CLINICS IN DEVELOPMENTAL MEDICINE NO. 92
ULTRASOUND OF THE INFANT BRAIN

Clinics in Developmental Medicine No. 92

ULTRASOUND OF THE INFANT BRAIN

MALCOLM I. LEVENE
JONATHAN L. WILLIAMS
CLAIRE-LISE FAWER

1985
Spastics International Medical Publications
OXFORD: Blackwell Scientific Publications Ltd.
PHILADELPHIA: J.B. Lippincott Co.

© 1985 Spastics International Medical Publications
5a Netherhall Gardens, London NW3 5RN

First published 1985

British Library Cataloguing in Publication Data

Levene, Malcolm I.
    Ultrasound of the Infant Brain.—Clinics in
    Developmental Medicine No. 92
    1. Ultrasonic encephalography   2. Infants
    —Diseases—Diagnosis
    I. Title   II. Williams, Jonathan L.
    III. Fawer, Claire-Lise   IV. Series
    618.92′8047543   RJ488.5.U47

ISBN 0-632-01327-3

Printed in Great Britain at The Lavenham Press Ltd., Lavenham, Suffolk

CONTENTS

AUTHORS' APPOINTMENTS

MALCOLM I. LEVENE — Senior Lecturer, Honorary Consultant Paediatrician, Leicester University Medical School; formerly of Hammersmith Hospital, London.

JONATHAN L. WILLIAMS — Paediatric Radiologist, University of Florida School of Medicine, Gainesville; formerly of St. Christopher's Hospital for Children, Philadelphia.

CLAIRE-LISE FAWER — Research Fellow, Neonatal Unit, Department of Paediatrics, University of Lausanne, Switzerland.

FOREWORD

During the last decade, ultrasound examination of the infant brain has changed from a research tool available at a few centres to an almost routine investigative procedure in most neonatal intensive care units. This wide acceptance is based upon its portability, safety, excellent correlation with pathological specimens and considerable technological advances in equipment. We have seen cranial ultrasound grow from its modest beginnings to become an almost indispensible routine technique, and have drawn upon our collective experience to produce this book.

We represent the clinical and radiological disciplines using ultrasound for cranial examinations, and the international flavour of our backgrounds allows us to view the subject across speciality or national boundaries. Our different trainings and backgrounds have helped to convince us of the value of a combined approach to neonatal cranial ultrasonography. The clinical approach has prompted us to ask questions of ultrasound with particular reference to periventricular haemorrhage and its sequelae. The paediatric radiologist with his perspective of imaging techniques can guide the clinician to the most appropriate use of ultrasound. We hope that this combined approach will be of value to the reader.

This book is written as a general text for the clinical or imaging ultrasonographer. Complete discussions of all intracranial diseases are beyond our scope. References have been chosen from an abundant literature and are not intended to be exhaustive. Our aim is to share our combined experience and knowledge with the more accomplished investigator, while at the same time encouraging and directing the novice. Our common goal is to improve the care and management of the newborn infant.

ACKNOWLEDGEMENTS

In the preparation of this book we have relied heavily on the encouragement and support of our colleagues and mentors. We wish to thank Professor André Calame, Dr. Marie Capitanio, Professor Victor Dubowitz, Professor Hamish Simpson, Dr. Jonathan Wigglesworth and Dr. Clyde Williams for allowing us time to develop experience and for guiding our activities. Our appreciation is extended to Drs. Barry Goldberg, Sidney Leeman and Arnold Shkolnik for encouragement, advice and implanting a sense of excitement with ultrasound techniques.

We are grateful to those clinicians who allowed us to reproduce their illustrations, including Drs. A. Anderegg, N. Archer, M. Biliski, L. de Vries, M. Flouck, R. Jones, E. Perentes and John Trounce. We also thank Mrs. Ruth George, Ms. Linda Pigott and Mrs. M. Marion for invaluable and excellent secretarial assistance. The illustrations have been prepared by the Departments of Illustration of the Leicester Royal Infirmary, University of Florida and CHUV, to whom we are most grateful. In particular Ms. Liz Faulkner, without whose help many of the illustrations would be of poorer quality.

We thank Drs. Henry Baird, Martin Bax and Aidan MacFarlane for enthusiastic support for this venture from the conception to completion; and to Edward Fenton for editorial assistance. Dr. Fawer was supported by the Swiss National Science Foundation.

This book is dedicated to our patients, from whom we have learned; and also to Helen, who would have been proud to see the results of our efforts.

1
PHYSICS AND INSTRUMENTATION

History of ultrasound

Early attempts to use returning echoes to image organs began in Austria in 1937. Further research was delayed by World War II, but this period saw the development of 'sonar' and 'asdic' for military purposes. During the late 1940s, echoes from deep tissue interfaces were demonstrated in humans, utilising the principles of sonar refined during the war years. The technique of compounding or summating several 'sweeps' of the transducer was performed with the patient inside a water-filled B29 gun-turret (Holmes 1980). Commercial metal-stress detectors were then modified in Glasgow to develop devices to image the pelvis and the gravid uterus in cross-section. Echocardiography was developing rapidly in Malmo, Dusseldorf and London, while ophthalmic ultrasonography was demonstrating foreign bodies in and around the optic globe.

In Lund, Sweden, in 1952, ultrasound imaging was initiated in humans with the demonstration of echoes originating from the midline structures of a normal child. Soon afterwards, a shift of these midline echoes was found in another child who had a frontal haematoma. Refinements in the technique of fixed single-crystal imaging occurred over the next decade (Tenner 1975); the use of ultrasound in intracranial studies did not become widespread until the development of articulated arm devices, grey scale and real-time units.

The physics of ultrasound

Sound travels through liquids, solids and gasses in waves of *compression* and *rarefaction* of the space between molecules (Steidley 1977, Powis 1978). The ability of these alternating waves to pass through physical materials is dependent upon the acoustic 'density' of that material. For example, the energy required to deform air is considerably less than that necessary to cause a thick steel bar to vibrate. Denser substances thus resist sound-wave transmission and exhibit relatively higher *acoustical impedance*.

Another physical property of sound travelling through matter is the relationship of the speed of sound transmission (v), the distance between serial molecule compressions (λ) and the vibrations per second or frequency (f). This relationship is written: $v = \lambda f$ (Fig. 1.1). For most biological tissues, velocity (v) does not change significantly; therefore if the wavelength (λ) is increased, the frequency (f) must decrease (Avecilla 1979).

As sound-waves pass through tissues, energy is lost to the adjacent regions in the form of increased molecular motion or heat. Energy loss from the sound-wave also occurs as a result of the compactness of the molecular particles. Tightly packed particles may not transmit coherently because the vibrations may get out of synchronization. In addition, the small zones of rarefaction and compression used

1

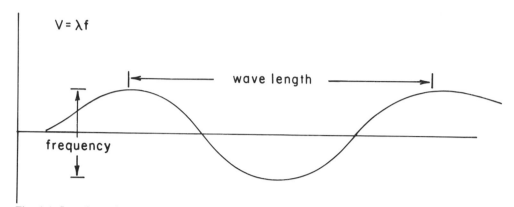

Fig. 1.1. Interdependence of velocity, wavelength and frequency. As velocity of sound transmission through biological materials is relatively fixed, an increase in sound-wave frequency requires a decrease in wavelength.

in diagnostic ultrasound are not well transmitted if the moving particles are far apart in space, as in a gas. This group of degrading properties is called *attenuation*.

The source of sound activity in an ultrasound device is the *piezo-electric transducer*. Certain natural crystals have the property of generating minute electrical impulses if their lattice is deformed by mechanical means. In addition, when a small electrical impulse is applied to this same crystal, it will expand or contract depending upon the polarity of the electrical charge. Thus, this special material can emit sound-waves and also respond electrically to returning mechanical deforming forces (Fig. 1.2). Cultured crystals of lead zirconate and lead titanate (PZT crystals) are now used instead of the naturally occurring quartz. Each crystal vibrates with a specific and fixed frequency. At diagnostic ultrasound levels, this frequency range includes crystals that oscillate from 2.5 million cycles per second (2.5 megahertz) up to 10 million cycles per second (10 megahertz). The human ear can respond to sound frequencies in the range of 20 to 20,000 cycles per second.

When an ultrasound wave from a transducer has entered biological tissue, the direction of the main wave front is influenced by that tissue (Sommer 1979). An echo is produced when the wave strikes the interface of two regions with differing acoustical impedance. If all the sound energy is returned to the transducer, complete reflection has occurred. A more likely situation is that the primary beam strikes the interface obliquely. This results in some of the sound energy returning to the transducer, some passing through the interface, and some deflected at an oblique angle. These possible interactions at the acoustical interface are referred to as *reflection*, and *refraction* (Fig. 1.3).

In order to produce an ultrasound image, the distance from the reflecting interface to the transducer must be computed. This can be done by knowing the speed of sound in soft tissue (approximately 1540 m/sec) and by measuring the time required for the echo to strike the transducer. A simple calculation with these data will reveal the distance of the reflecting object.

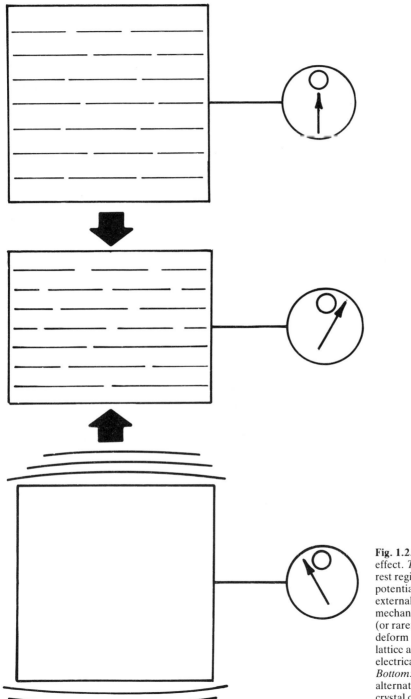

Fig. 1.2. Piezo-electric effect. *Top:* a crystal at rest registers zero potential. *Centre:* externally applied mechanical compressive (or rarefraction) forces deform the crystal lattice and produce an electrical potential. *Bottom:* applying an alternating current to crystal causes lattice to expand and contract.

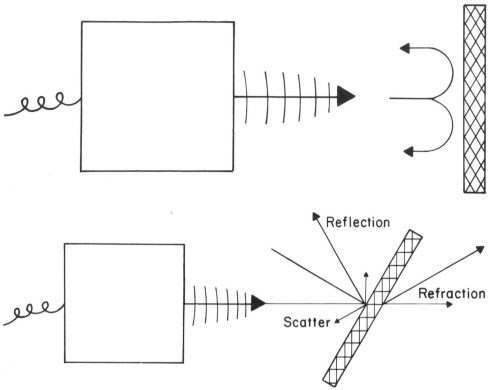

Fig. 1.3. Reflection and refraction. *Top:* when acoustic interface is perpendicular to the sound-wave, complete reflection occurs. *Bottom:* when interface is oblique, a portion of the wave is reflected, some passes through but at a slightly different angle, and some is scattered.

The width of the crystal-generated sound-beam is directly proportional to the diameter of the transducer face. However, because of tissue interaction and internal beam disharmony, distal flaring occurs. This flaring introduces some error in object size estimations. For example, when a near reflecting object partly obliterates the full diameter of the beam, its size appears to match the transducer face. If a more distant object also partly reflects the beam width, its size appears to be larger than the near object. In fact, if the distal object is the same size as the near one, it only appears to be larger because of flaring of the more distal sound-beam (Fig. 1.4). This is referred to as *lateral resolution* and is dependent upon the width of the beam in the near (Fresnel) or far (Fraunhofer) field. *Axial resolution* refers to how small and how close two reflecting objects can be and still be seen as separate objects, independent of their location along the axis of the beam.

In order to compensate for this flaring of the far field, a focusing lens can be placed in front of the transducer. A more popular system is to use a concave crystal face, and such converging crystals are described as *internally focused*.

4

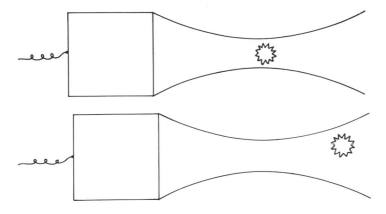

Fig. 1.4. Lateral resolution. *Top:* reflecting interface in near or focused zone is in sharp focus. *Bottom:* divergence of distal beam (far zone) produces fuzzy margins, and object appears slightly larger.

The difficulties produced by artefacts are clearly explained by Laing (1982) and Laing and Kurtz (1983).

Instrumentation

A transducer crystal generates a single pencil-like wave of ultrasound energy. Placing this single element on tissue produces echoes only from that core of tissue. The size of the imaged field is roughly that of the crystal diameter. In order to image larger volumes of tissue, such as a liver, multiple 'cores' are projected sequentially on a monitor, while the transducer is moved over the organ. On this device, called a persistence-scope, each core of echoes remains on a television screen until the entire image field is electronically erased. Connecting the transducer through an articulated arm device to a position-sensing computer allows imaging of planar tissue volumes (Hagen-Ansert 1978). This manual movement of the transducer produces *static images*.

Single-crystal transducers can be mechanically wobbled or rocked within a housing. This produces a wedge-shaped image of tissue rather than a pencil-shaped core. A rotating wheel with several transducers attached to it will produce a similar wedge-shaped image. Successive images are placed on a television monitor and rapidly erased, producing an image in *real-time*. Respiration effect, vascular pulsation, peristalsis and other organ motion is clearly displayed. There is no time delay from event to observation. Frame rates of about 60/second remove flicker, or 'image stepping' which will occur at rates of 15 to 30/second.

A multiple series of crystals may be placed side by side within a housing. Such *linear array* transducers image larger volumes of tissue; 64 element units are common. Varying the activation sequence of these multi-element devices will result in angled or sectored views. These electronically controlled devices are called *phased linear arrays*.

Another transducer configuration relies upon no contact with the skin surface. The transducers are placed within a water-filled housing, covered by a flexible membrane upon which the patient lies. These multiple finely focused transducers are controlled electronically from a remote console. This is the *automated water*

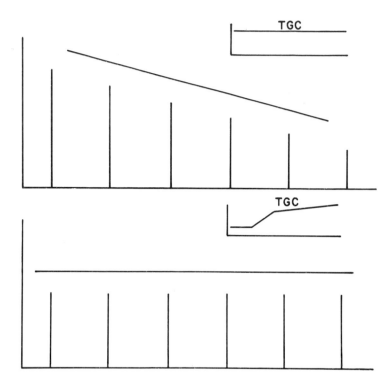

Fig. 1.5. Time gain compensation. *Top:* echoes from reflectors near transducer are stronger while those more distant are weaker due to attenuation and scatter. *Bottom:* electronic near-field suppression and far-field enhancement produces more even echo display.

path configuration. Images from this device are only static.

As a result of tissue attenuation of the sound-beam, selective enhancement of the faint echoes from deeper interfaces is desirable. This is performed by way of an electronic circuit which suppresses the relatively strong near echoes (short time of travel) while increasing the observed echo responses (gain) from those acoustic interfaces at a greater depth from the transducer. Adjustment of this time-gain compensation (TGC) curve is dependent upon the image seen on the monitor (Fig. 1.5).

A pulse generator produces the electronic impulses that activate the sending mode in the transducer (Sarti and Sample 1980). Matching or synchronisation with the other components of the device is also a function of the pulse generator. Returning echoes are received by the transducer, and amplified symmetrically to preserve relative amplitudes. The receiver or demodulator then filters out extraneous electronic noise and computes the position of each echo. These signals are then delivered to a television screen or monitor which prints out the final image. A permanent record may then be extracted from the monitor image and placed on standard videotape, photographed, or etched on heat-sensitive paper.

Biological effects of diagnostic ultrasound

The widespread application and frequent use of ultrasound imaging has caused concern about the safety of this technique (Lele 1979, Martin 1984). Echoes may be produced in a continuous fashion but most imaging is performed utilising an intermittent pulse. Almost all commercial devices generate sound-pulses relatively infrequently, and the transducers are in the receiving or 'listening' state 99.9 per cent of the operational time. Quality control in commercial production allows maximal transducer output to be in the range of 1 to 50 mw/cm^2. This is about 100 times less than the energy output required for ultrasound diathermy treatment.

Known biological effects may be divided into three general classes: heat generation, cavitation and vibration effects on large particles (Baker and Dalrymple 1978).

Sound-waves are a form of mechanical energy, and attenuation by tissues causes a reduction in the power of the sound-beam. Direct absorption of some portion of this energy is transmitted to tissue as heat. In diagnostic power ranges, no heating of small tissue volumes has been measured. Focal cellular heating effects may occur but have not been consistently measured nor their effects demonstrated.

Cavitation refers to the formation of microbubbles in biological solutions. The waves of compression and rarefaction in turn set up currents in fluids or 'microstreaming'. Microbubbles and microstreaming produce focal regions of fluid shear, which may mechanically distort cell membranes and organelles. However, cavitation occurs with much longer exposure times and with considerably wider pulse-sequences than those found in diagnostic ultrasound.

Mechanical vibration effects on macromolecules such as DNA are possible. Some experimental work has demonstrated changes in cell membrane morphology (Liebeskind et al. 1981), suggested transient chromosome disruption, and shown some growth-distortion of cells in tissue culture (Liebeskind et al. 1979). No specific oncogenic effects have been shown. Other careful experimental studies have not confirmed these findings, and found little or no demonstrable effect.

Evaluation of the risks and benefits to the patient are still important, but most investigators agree that no significant adverse clinical effects of diagnostic ultrasound imaging on humans are yet known (AIUM 1984). The biological effect from performing multiple repeated examinations over a short period of time is less certain. Nevertheless, there is a high safety factor when using ultrasound imaging compared with ionizing radiation imaging techniques.

REFERENCES

A.I.U.M. (1984) 'Statement on clinical safety.' *Journal of Ultrasound in Medicine,* **3**, R-10.

Avecilla, L. S. (1979) 'The physics and instrumentation of diagnostic ultrasound: a review, part I.' *Medical Ultrasound,* **3**, 11-15.

Baker, M. L., Dalrymple, G. V. (1978) 'Biological effects of diagnostic ultrasound: a review.' *Radiology,* **126**, 479-483.

Hagen-Ansert, S. L. (1978) *Textbook of Diagnostic Ultrasonography.* St. Louis: Mosby. pp. 2-25.

Holmes, J. H. (1980) 'Diagnostic ultrasound during the early years of A.I.U.M.' *Journal of Clinical Ultrasound,* **8**, 299-308.

Laing, F. C. (1983) 'Commonly encountered artifacts in clinical ultrasound.' *Seminars in Ultrasound,* **4**, 27-43.

—— Kurtz, A. B. (1982) 'The importance of ultrasonic sidelobe artifacts.' *Radiology,* **145**, 763-768.

Lele, P. P. (1979) 'Safety and potential hazards in the current applications of ultrasound in obstetrics and gynecology.' *Ultrasound in Medicine and Biology,* **5**, 307-320.

Liebeskind, D., Bases, R., Elequin, F., Neubort, S., Leifer, R., Goldberg, R., Koenigsberg, M. (1979) 'Diagnostic ultrasound: effects on the DNA and growth patterns of animal cells.' *Radiology,* **131,** 177-184.

—— —— Koenigsberg, M., Koss, L., Raventos, C. (1981) 'Morphological changes in the surface characteristics of cultured cells after exposure to diagnostic ultrasound.' *Radiology,* **138,** 419-423.

Martin, A. O. (1984) 'Can ultrasound cause genetic damage?' *Journal of Clinical Ultrasound,* **12,** 11-20.

Powis, R. L. (1978) *Ultrasound Physics for the Fun of it.* Unirad Corporation.

Sarti, D. A., Sample, W. F. (Eds.) (1980) *Diagnostic Ultrasound: Text and Cases.* Boston: Hall. pp. 1-21.

Sommer, F. G., Filly, R. A., Minton, M. J. (1979) 'Acoustic shadowing due to refractive and reflective effects.' *American Journal of Roentgenology,* **132,** 973-977.

Steidley, K. D. (1977) 'An introduction to the physics of diagnostic ultrasound.' *Applied Radiology,* (March/April), 155-170.

Tenner, M. S., Wodraska, G. M. (1975) *Diagnostic Ultrasound in Neurology.* New York: Wiley.

2
SCANNING TECHNIQUES AND NORMAL ANATOMY

Techniques of scanning
Cranial ultrasound scans are commonly performed in coronal and sagittal planes, using the anterior fontanelle as an acoustic window (Babcock *et al.* 1980, Grant *et al.* 1980, Babcock and Han 1981, Levene *et al.* 1981, Pigadas *et al.* 1981, Shuman *et al.* 1981, Couture and Cadier 1983, Cremin *et al.* 1983). These imaging planes are shown in Figure 2.1. An additional scan series can be obtained in the axial plane by placing the transducer laterally on the scalp parallel to the canthohelical line, as shown in Figure 2.2 (Kossoff *et al.* 1974, Johnson *et al.* 1979).

Coronal planes
The transducer is oriented in the coronal plane after palpation of the anterior fontanelle and is then angled from front to back. Several sequential sections are obtained:
A. anterior coronal section through the frontal lobes
B. anterior coronal section through the frontal horns
C. coronal section at the level of the foramen of Monro and the third ventricle
D. coronal section through the bodies of the lateral ventricles
E. coronal section through the trigone of the lateral ventricles
F. posterior coronal section through the occipital lobes.

Sagittal planes
The transducer is turned through 90 degrees from the position used for the coronal sections. Each hemisphere is visualised by angling the ultrasound beam to the left and right of the midline toward the Sylvian fissures. The following sections are obtained:
G. midline section including the corpus callosum, third and fourth ventricles and the cerebellar vermis
H. parasagittal section through the lateral venticle, angling the transducer 10 to 20 degrees posteriorly to allow for the divergence of the occipital horns (Fig. 2.1). Multiple parasagittal sections may be needed to completely visualise the lateral ventricles
I. extreme parasagittal sections through the insulae.

Axial planes
Two sections are usually obtained:
J. axial section through the cerebral peduncles
K. axial section at the level of the bodies of the lateral ventricles.

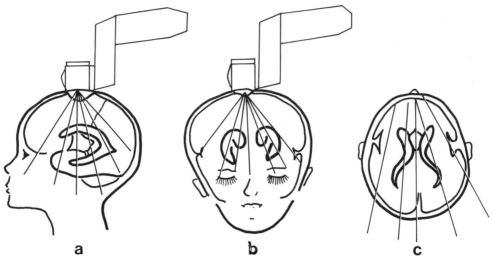

Fig. 2.1. Schematic diagrams to illustrate the planes in which scanning can be performed through anterior fontanelle. **(a)** Coronal. **(b and c)** Sagittal.

Image orientation

Coronal planes are displayed with the patient's right on the right side of the image. Sagittal planes are displayed with the patient's face to the left side of the image and the right or left hemispheres are appropriately labelled. Unless indicated otherwise, the scans show the patient's face to the left.

Ultrasound and anatomical descriptions of cerebral structure
Skull, falx and tentorium

The bones of the skull appear as thick and hyperechoic lines.

CORONAL PLANES

In the anterior cranial fossa, the lateral margins consist of the temporal and frontal bones, and the ethmoid bones make up its floor (Fig. 2.3). The orbits and globes

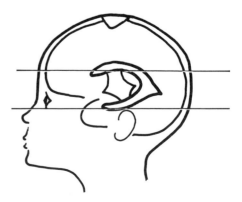

Fig. 2.2. Schematic diagram to illustrate planes for axial scans through temporoparietal bone.

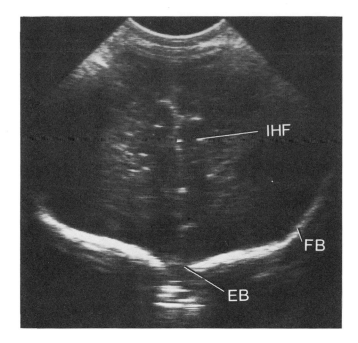

Fig. 2.3. Coronal scan through anterior cranial fossa. Frontal bone (FB), ethmoid bone (EB), interhemispheric fissure (IHF).

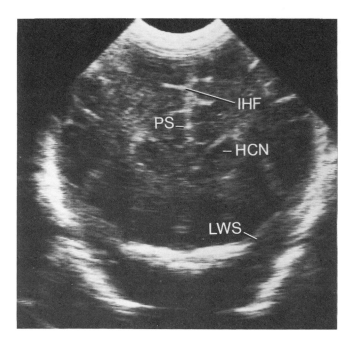

Fig. 2.4. Coronal scan through sphenoid bone. Interhemispheric fissure (IHF), pericallosal sulci (PS), lesser wings of sphenoid (LWS), head of caudate nucleus (HCN).

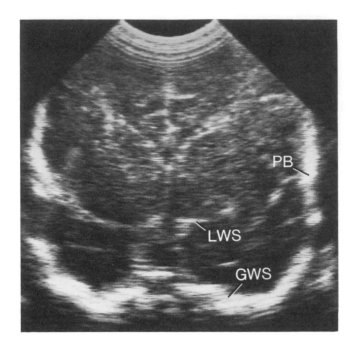

Fig. 2.5. Coronal scan through middle cranial fossa at level of sphenoid bone. Parietal bone (PB), lesser wings of sphenoid (LWS), greater wings of sphenoid (GWS).

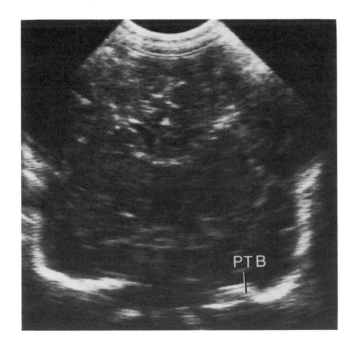

Fig. 2.6. Coronal scan through middle cranial fossa at level of petrous temporal bone (PTB).

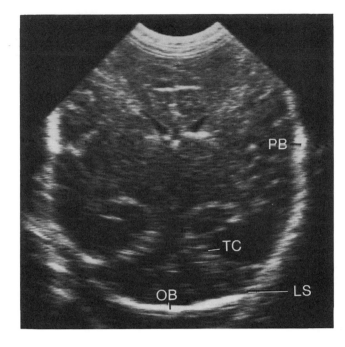

Fig. 2.7. Coronal scan through posterior cranial fossa. Parietal bone (PB), occipital bone (OB), lamboid sutures (LS), tentorium cerebelli (TC).

may be seen. Prominent reflections from the cingulate sulci extend laterally (Fig. 2.4). The interhemispheric fissure and the falx cerebri produce an echogenic midline structure separating the hemispheres. It is possible to identify the falx only when the interhemispheric fissure is enlarged.

In the middle cranial fossa, the parietal bones form the lateral limits. The middle portion of its floor is made up by the sphenoid bone which is strongly echogenic. If the transducer is then angled slightly posteriorly, the wings of the sphenoid are noted on either side and appear as horizontal echogenic thin lines (Figs. 2.4 and 2.5). The interhemispheric fissure forms a vertical echogenic line with its base resting on the corpus callosum. Further small posterior movement visualises the petrous temporal bones (Fig. 2.6).

The lateral margins of the posterior cranial fossa are formed by the parietal bones which are separated posteriorly from the occipital bone by the lamboid sutures. The posterior fossa is limited inferiorly by the leaves of the tentorium cerebelli, which appear as two oblique echogenic lines with their bases on the occipital bones (Fig. 2.7).

SAGITTAL PLANES

In the midline image the vault is formed anteriorly by the frontal bones. The sphenoid bone forms the anterior margin of the middle cranial fossa with the sella turcica and clivus forming the posterior margin. The posterior cranial fossa is limited by the occipital bone (Fig. 2.8).

On parasagittal sections the floor of the middle cranial fossa consists of echoes

13

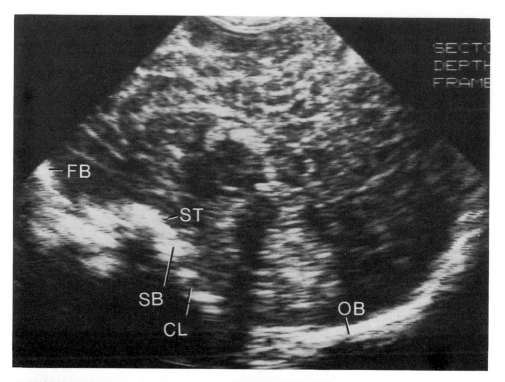

Fig. 2.8. *(above):* midline
sagittal scan. Frontal bone
(FB), sphenoid bone (SB),
sella turcica (ST), clivus
(Cl), occipital bone (OB).

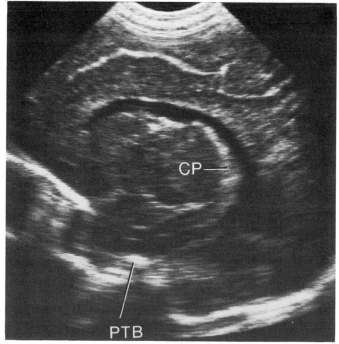

Fig. 2.9. *(left):* parasagittal
scan. Petrous temporal
bone (PTB), choroid
plexus (CP).

14

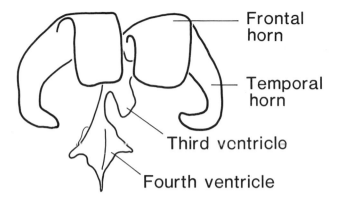

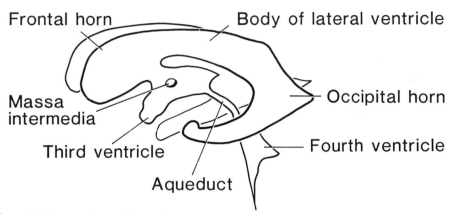

Fig. 2.10. Diagram of ventricular system.

originating from the petrous temporal bones (Fig. 2.9). The tentorium cerebelli is not visualised in this plane because of its oblique orientation.

The ventricular system
The ventricular system includes two lateral ventricles, the third and fourth ventricle. They communicate with each other and with the subarachnoid spaces. In the term newborn infant they are often quite difficult to visualise. The lateral ventricles form the largest cavities of the ventricular system and are situated in the lower medial portion of each cerebral hemisphere. They are separated by the septum pellucidum. Each lateral ventricle consists of a body and three horns (Fig. 2.10). The body extends from the foramen of Monro to the trigone and is triangular in coronal section with its apex pointing medially and downward. The frontal horn passes forward and laterally and then dips slightly downward into the frontal lobe. Its anterior portion curves around the head of the caudate nucleus. The occipital horn extends laterally and posteriorly into the occipital lobe, and has a variable

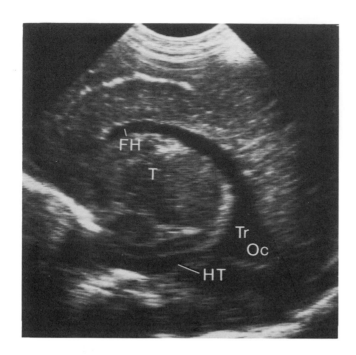

Fig. 2.11. Parasagittal scan showing lateral ventricles. Frontal horn (FH), occipital horn (Oc), temporal horn (HT), trigone (Tr), thalamus (T).

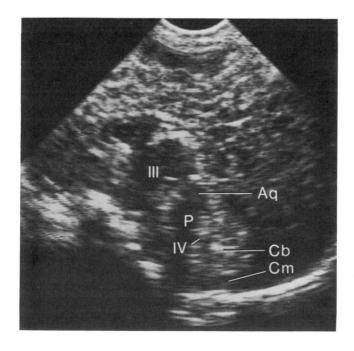

Fig. 2.12. Midline sagittal scan. Third ventricle (III), aqueduct of Sylvius (Aq), fourth ventricle (IV), cerebellum (Cb), pons (P), cisterna magna (CM).

16

triangular shape. The temporal horn curves laterally around the thalamus, and then extends downward and forward within the temporal lobe. The trigone is situated at the junction of temporal, frontal and occipital horns (Fig. 2.11).

The ventricular cavities represent the main echo-free landmarks within the brain. Variations in their size and position aid the detection and description of cerebral malformations. The third ventricle is a thin, centrally located cleft which lies between the two thalami. It communicates with the lateral ventricles through the foramina of Monro, and with the fourth ventricle *via* the aqueduct of Sylvius. The supra-optic and infundibular recesses give its characteristic triangular shape on sagittal scan. The third ventricle is narrow and is frequently not seen on coronal section.

The aqueduct of Sylvius is a slender channel, and is rarely seen on ultrasound examination (Fig. 2.12). The fourth ventricle is a small cavity with a rhomboid shape. Its superior limit is the aqueduct of Sylvius and its inferior limit is the central canal of the medulla oblongata. It appears as a small anechoic triangle with its apex directed into the cerebellar vermis (Fig. 2.12).

Cavum septi pellucidi and cavum vergae
A cavity between the leaves of the septum pellucidum is commonly seen and represents incomplete fusion. This is a normal variation in newborn infants. The cavum septi pellucidi and cavum vergae are the same structure, the former located anteriorly to the columns of the fornices and the latter extends posteriorly (Fig. 2.13). These cavities vary considerably in size (Farrugia and Babcock 1981), and are almost always present in premature infants (Grant *et al.* 1980). Posterior obliteration occurs initially, so the cavum vergae is usually absent in term neonates. This space usually does not communicate with the ventricular system (Shaw and Alvord 1969). Care should be taken not to confuse these structures with the third ventricle.

Choroid plexus
The choroid plexus lies on the floor of the lateral ventricle. It takes a semi-circular course from the temporal horn around the thalamus and into the body of the lateral ventricle. It almost reaches the foramen of Monro. It is narrow in the temporal horn and becomes more bulbous in the trigone area. Choroid plexi are also found posteriorly along the roof of the third and fourth ventricles. The choroid plexus appears as a hyperechoic structure, and represents one of the most prominent landmarks in the neonatal brain. Their highly echogenic appearance is due to their configuration and the close vicinity of fluid-filled spaces. The choroid plexus consists of multiple vascular villi which produce numerous small interfaces that are responsible for its echogenicity (Fig. 2.9).

Cerebellum
In coronal scans the cerebellum lies below the tentorium, and is an echogenic structure within the posterior fossa. In the full-term infant the cerebellar vermis is a particularly reflective structure, and on coronal scan is seen in the midline within

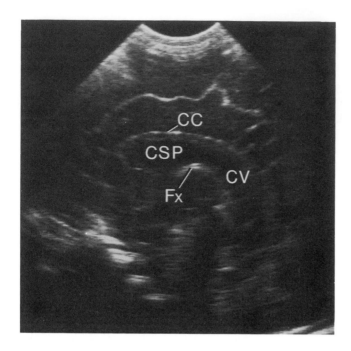

Fig. 2.13. Midline sagittal scan. Cavum septi pellucidi (CSP), cavum vergae (CV), fornix (Fx), corpus callosum (CC).

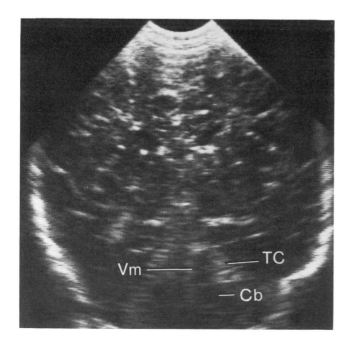

Fig. 2.14. Coronal scan through the posterior cranial fossa. Cerebellum (Cb), tentorium cerebelli (TC), vermis (Vm).

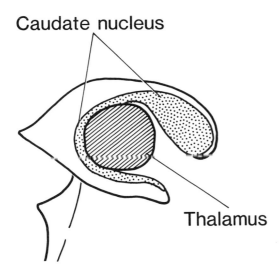

Caudate nucleus

Thalamus

Fig. 2.15. Diagram of basal nuclei.

the cerebellum (Fig. 2.14). On midline sagittal scan, the cerebellum is pear-shaped and situated behind the pons and the fourth ventricle (Fig. 2.12). Goodwin and Quisling (1983) have studied the cisterna magna by ultrasound and provided measurements of this structure and the normal fourth ventricle.

Basal nuclei
The caudate nucleus is an area of grey matter applied to the infero-lateral wall of the lateral ventricle. The head of the caudate nucleus lies beneath the frontal horn, anterior to the foramen of Monro. The body then extends posteriorly along the floor of the lateral ventricle. The tail lies in the roof of the temporal horn. The head of the caudate is seen on both coronal (Fig. 2.4) and sagittal planes (Fig. 2.15).

The thalamic nuclei consist of two symmetrical ovoid structures situated on either side of the septum pellucidum and the third ventricle. They are connected to each other by the massa intermedia through the body of the third ventricle. Their lateral margins lie adjacent to the internal capsule. On coronal and parasagittal sections they appear as discrete structures of relatively low echodensity (Fig. 2.11). The lenticular nucleus, claustrum and the internal capsule lie between the thalamus and the insula. It is not possible to differentiate these structures because of their similar echodensity.

Vascular supply of the brain
Arteries appear as bright pulsatile reflections when seen with real-time ultrasound (Fig. 2.16). Venous channels are poorly seen. The internal carotid artery supplies the brain lying in the anterior and middle cranial fossae, whilst the vertebral artery supplies the posterior fossa contents.

The circle of Willis is an arterial ring surrounding the optic chiasma and pituitary stalk. It is recognised by its prominent vascular pulsations in the base of

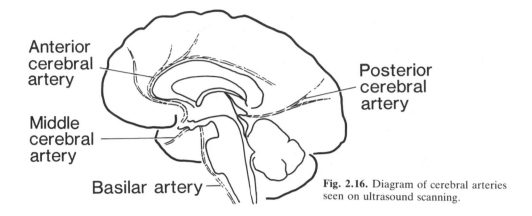

Anterior cerebral artery

Posterior cerebral artery

Middle cerebral artery

Basilar artery

Fig. 2.16. Diagram of cerebral arteries seen on ultrasound scanning.

the middle cranial fossa on both coronal and sagittal sections. The anterior cerebral artery arises from the anterior portion of the circle of Willis, and both branches extend anterior and superior to the rostrum of the corpus callosum. The anterior cerebral artery then gives off a branch which runs above the corpus callosum and is seen on coronal and sagittal sections. Figure 2.17 shows the arteries recognised on coronal scans.

The middle cerebral artery arises from the internal carotid and is seen laterally as pulsatile echoes. The main branch of the middle cerebral artery lies in the Sylvian fissure, and this represents a constant and distinctive pulsating landmark. Other pulsating vessels may be seen as focal echodensities in sulci and fissures.

Ultrasound sections

Coronal planes

These sections are described separately as shown in Figure 2.18.

ANTERIOR CORONAL SECTION THROUGH THE FRONTAL LOBES (Image A) (Fig. 2.19). In this plane, several structures are seen. The interhemispheric fissure and the falx cerebri form a thin vertical echogenic line bisecting the anterior cranial fossa above the orbits. The anterior lobes may appear fairly echogenic in their central part especially in premature infants. This feature is physiological and should not be mistaken for a pathological process.

ANTERIOR CORONAL SECTION THROUGH THE FRONTAL HORNS (Image B) (Fig. 2.20). The frontal horns form two triangular echo-free areas. The interhemispheric fissure and falx form the midline and extend to the corpus callosum. The corpus callosum appears as a relatively anechoic horizontal band, limited above by the base of the interhemispheric fissure and below by the roof of both lateral ventricles and septum pellucidum. The head of the caudate nucleus is seen as a slightly echogenic structure beneath the frontal horns. The cerebral parenchyma in the very immature brain appears as a poorly echogenic structure.

CORONAL SECTION AT THE LEVEL OF THE FORAMEN OF MONRO (Image C) (Fig. 2.21). At this level the lateral ventricles appear as anechoic cavities. In the term infant

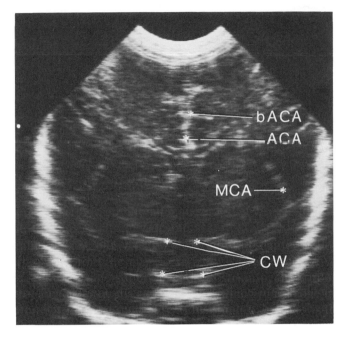

Fig. 2.17. Coronal scan through middle cranial fossa showing the position of arteries. Temporal branch of middle cerebral artery (MCA), anterior cerebral artery (ACA), branches of anterior cerebral artery (bACA), vessels of circle of Willis (CW).

they are sometimes difficult to identify. The foramen of Monro is visualised by moving the transducer forward and backward and appears as an anechoic structure connecting both lateral ventricles with the third ventricle. The choroid plexi of the lateral and third ventricles form a hyperechoic midline structure as they fuse at the foramen of Monro. This appearance should not be confused with haemorrhage. Other important structures include the corpus callosum, the caudate nucleus and the thalamic nucleus. The Sylvian fissures are seen as lateral symmetrical thin echogenic lines with a characteristic 'Y' shape, containing the pulsating echoes of the temporal branches of the middle cerebral arteries. In the cerebral parenchyma, the hippocampal gyri (temporal lobes) and the cingulate gyri (frontal lobes) can be differentiated. The cavum septi pellucidi may vary in size and shape and appear as a triangular cavity between the lateral ventricles. The third ventricle is often not clearly seen. It forms a thin cleft between the thalami with indistinct lateral margins. If the third ventricle is dilated the massa intermedia is noted as an echogenic band crossing the ventricles.

CORONAL SECTION THROUGH THE BODIES OF THE LATERAL VENTRICLES (Image D) (Fig. 2.22).

This plane demonstrates the bodies of the lateral ventricles, the corpus callosum, the cavum septi pellucidi and the Sylvian fissures. On the floor of the lateral ventricles, highly echogenic structures represent the choroid plexus. The pons produces a vertical echogenic band located between the hippocampal gyri. In the middle cranial fossa the Sylvian fissures, caudate nuclei, basal ganglia and pulsations from the circle of Willis are seen. The hippocampi are of relatively low

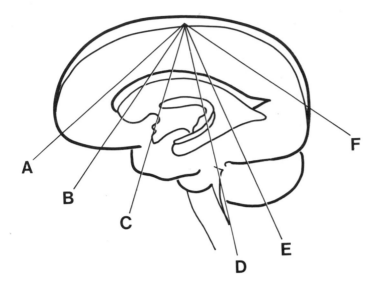

Fig. 2.18. Diagram of coronal planes referred to in text.

echogenicity. The posterior cranial fossa is visible in this plane and is limited superiorly by the bright echoes from the tentorium and cerebellum.

CORONAL SECTION THROUGH THE TRIGONE OF THE LATERAL VENTRICLES (Image E) (Fig. 2.23).

The main landmarks in this plane are the lateral ventricles which diverge. The ventricular cavity is partially or wholly filled by the echogenic choroid plexus. The interhemispheric fissure is seen with its inferior portion lying on the splenium of the corpus callosum. Within the posterior cranial fossa is the echogenic cerebellum, limited superiorly by the tentorium.

CORONAL SECTION THROUGH THE OCCIPITAL LOBES (Image F) (Fig. 2.24).

The interhemispheric fissure remains a thin, echogenic vertical line. The central part of the occipital lobes may appear moderately echogenic and this appearance is normal.

Sagittal sections

These sections are described separately as shown in Figure 2.25.

SAGITTAL MIDLINE SECTION (Image G) (Fig. 2.26).

The corpus callosum appears as an arcuate structure. The genu arches forward and downward, thinning out anteriorly to form the rostrum. Its midportion is relatively flat, and the thicker posterior portion (called the splenium) curves over the midbrain structures. The upper margin of the corpus callosum is marked by the pulsations from the pericallosal artery. The cingulate gyrus rests on the corpus callosum, and is limited by the cingulate sulcus which appears as a thin echogenic line.

Just beneath the corpus callosum the cavum septi pellucidi and vergae are seen, if present, as an echo-free cavity. They are quite often separated by a brightly echogenic band formed by the columns of the fornices and the choroid plexus of the

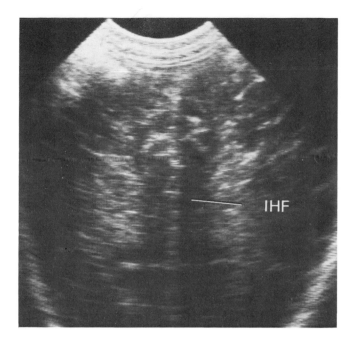

Fig. 2.19. Coronal section A. Interhemispheric fissure (IHF).

third ventricle. The third ventricle has a characteristic triangular shape, with the apex pointing towards the pituitary fossa. Its posterior wall contains the pineal gland and extends to the quadrigeminal plate. The pons and medulla are seen as vertical structures of low echodensity. The small echo-free triangular fourth ventricle lies posterior to the brainstem.

The posterior cranial fossa is occupied by the echogenic cerebellar vermis. The cerebral parenchyma is divided by the cingulate and parieto-occipital sulci and the calcarine fissure. Small extensions from the main sulci may be seen together with arterial pulsations from vessels within them.

PARASAGITTAL SECTION THROUGH THE LATERAL VENTRICLES (Image H) (Fig. 2.27). The transducer must be angled approximately 15 degrees laterally to obtain a complete image of the lateral ventricles as the occipital horns diverge away from the midline. The frontal, temporal and occipital horns, the trigone and the body of the lateral ventricles can be clearly seen. The choroid plexus forms an echogenic semi-circular structure around the thalamus and extends forward to the foramen of Monro. The foramen may be visualised as a small anechoic depression on the floor of the lateral ventricle. The glomus within the trigone is prominent.

Any area of increased echodensity located in the floor of the lateral ventricle, anterior to the foramen of Monro, should be considered as abnormal and may represent a haemorrhage. Fiske *et al.* (1981) described the normal appearance and configuration of the choroid plexus, and also discussed the differential diagnosis with haemorrhage in the subependymal plate (see Chapter 4). The thalamus and caudate nucleus are distinct structures, separated by a smooth echogenic line

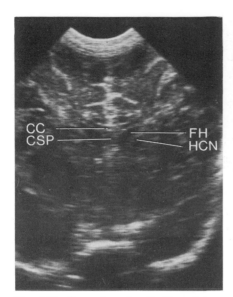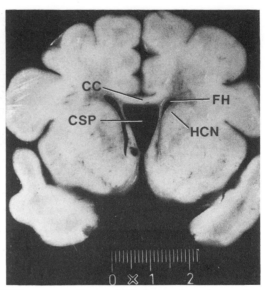

Fig. 2.20. Coronal section B. Frontal horns (FH), corpus callosum (CC), head of caudate nucleus (HCN), cavum septi pellucidi (CSP) is large on brain section and poorly seen on ultrasound image. Specimens are from different children.

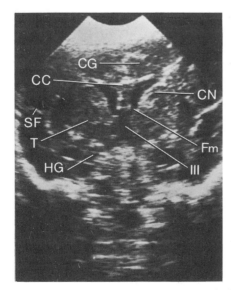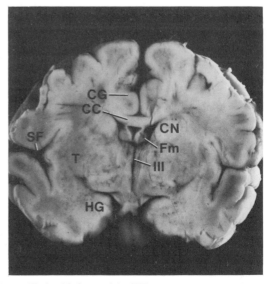

Fig. 2.21. Coronal section C. Foramen of Monro (Fm), third ventricle (III), corpus callosum (CC), caudate nucleus (CN), thalamus (T), Sylvian fissure (SF), hippocampal gyrus (HG), cingulate gyrus (CG).

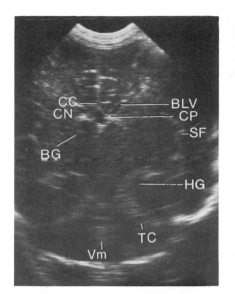
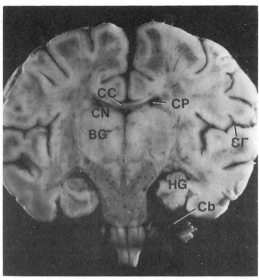

Fig. 2.22. Coronal section D. Body of lateral ventricle (BLV), corpus callosum (CC), Sylvian fissure (SF), choroid plexus (CP), hippocampal gyrus (HG), caudate nuclei (CN), basal ganglia (BG), tentorium cerebelli (TC), vermis (Vm).

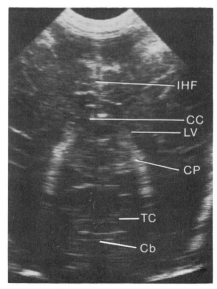
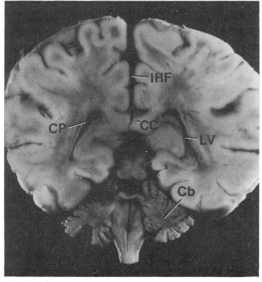

Fig. 2.23. Coronal section E. Lateral ventricle (LV), choroid plexus (CP), interhemispheric fissure (IHF), corpus callosum (CC), cerebellum (Cb), tentorium cerebelli (TC).

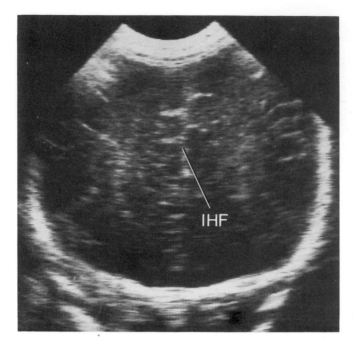

Fig. 2.24. Coronal section F. Interhemispheric fissure (IHF).

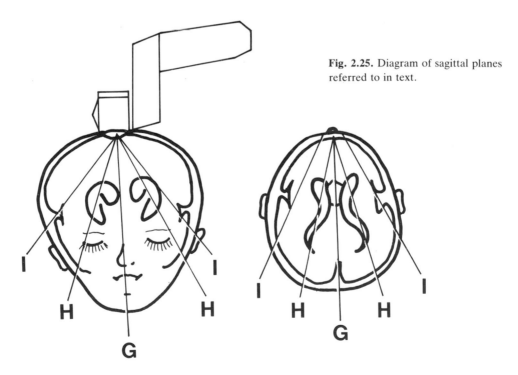

Fig. 2.25. Diagram of sagittal planes referred to in text.

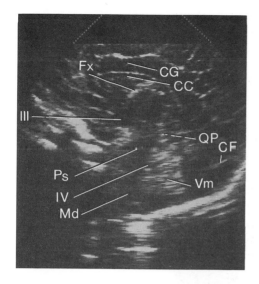

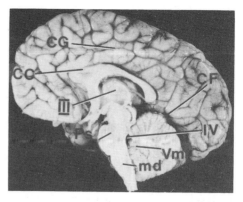

Fig. 2.26. Midline sagittal section G. Corpus callosum (CC), cingulate gyrus (CG), fornix (Fx), third ventricle (III), quadrigeminal plate (QP), pons (Ps), medulla (Md), fourth ventricle (IV), cerebellar vermis (Vm), calcarine fissure (CF).

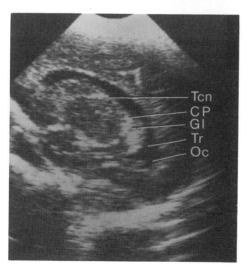

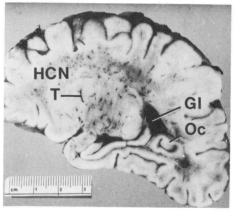

Fig. 2.27. Parasagittal section H. Occipital horn of lateral ventricle (Oc), trigone (Tr), choroid plexus (CP), glomus (Gl), thalamo-caudate notch (Tcn).

originating from the thalamo-caudate notch and the thalamo-striate vein.

PARASAGITTAL SECTION THROUGH THE INSULA (Image I) (Fig. 2.28).

The tortuous fissures of the operculum can be clearly seen in this plane. Pulsations from branches of the middle cerebral artery are present.

Axial sections

These sections are described in Figure 2.2.

AXIAL SECTION AT THE LEVEL OF THE CEREBRAL PEDUNCLES (Image J) (Fig. 2.29).

The cerebral peduncles are seen as hyperechogenic 'butterfly-shaped' structures. A

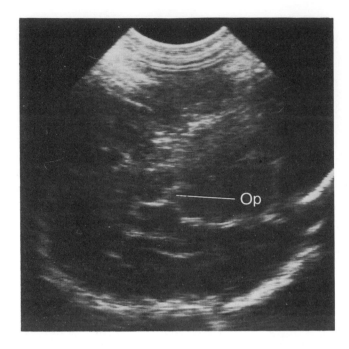

Fig. 2.28. Parasagittal section I. Operculum (Op). Posterior of brain is on left.

central echogenic spot is seen posteriorly and represents the aqueduct of Sylvius. Anterior to the peduncles, mamillary bodies are visible as two paired ovoid masses. The arteries at the base of the brain are seen as pulsatile echoes.

AXIAL SECTION AT THE LEVEL OF THE BODIES OF THE LATERAL VENTRICLES (Image κ) (Fig. 2.30).

The lateral walls of the bodies of the lateral ventricles appear as parallel echogenic lines diverging posteriorly. A straight midline echo originates from the interhemispheric fissure, falx cerebri and septum pellucidum. The opposite table of the skull is seen as a thick curved echo. The axial plane can be used to assess ventricular size when the anterior fontanelle is closed.

The axial sections correspond to the classical computed tomographic images. The ultrasound approach for the axial views is now rarely used, as coronal and parasagittal planes through the anterior fontanelle permit excellent definition of intracranial anatomy.

Development of the central nervous system

Cerebral development

During the first weeks of intra-uterine life, the neural tube closes and the cephalic pole divides into five parts: the telencephalon (cerebral hemispheres), diencephalon (thalamic structures), mesencephalon (midbrain), metencephalon (cerebellum) and myelencephalon (medulla). These structures are differentiated by 10 weeks. From the 10th week the ventricular cavity is filled by a proliferating choroid plexus. This appears initially in the fourth ventricle, then in the third, and finally in the

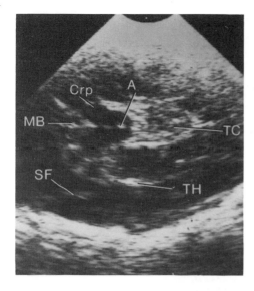

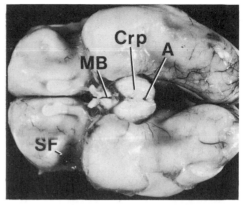

Fig. 2.29. Axial section J. Cerebral peduncles (Crp), aqueduct of Sylvius (A), mamillary bodies (MB), tentorium cerebelli (TC), Sylvian fissure (SF), temporal horn (TH). Posterior on right of scan.

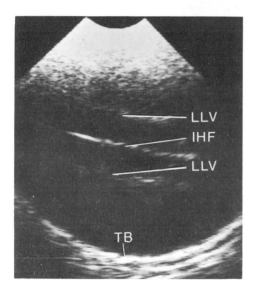

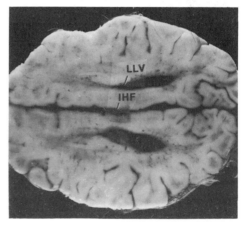

Fig. 2.30. Axial section K. Lateral walls of body of lateral ventricle (LLV), interhemispheric fissure (IHF), temporal bone (TB). Posterior on right of scan.

lateral ventricles (Fig. 2.31).

The increasing volume of the cerebral hemispheres is associated with progressive development of the sulci. Between the 24th and 28th weeks, the large primary sulci become deeper and more clearly defined. The posterior margins of the Sylvian fissure approximate due to the parallel development of the parietal and temporal lobes. At 28 weeks the calloso-marginal sulcus is present. The Sylvian fissure may still be open (Fig. 2.32), closing with the development of the frontal, parietal and temporal lobes. The complete development of the operculum covers

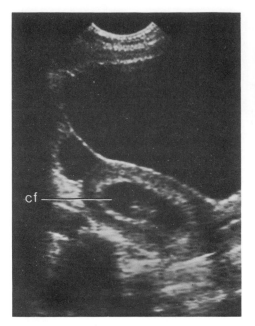

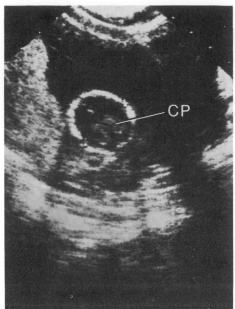

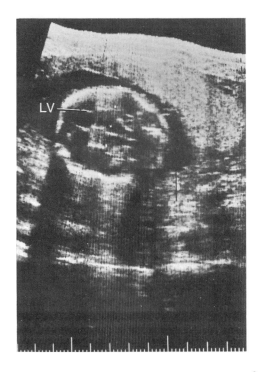

Fig. 2.31. Antepartum ultrasound scans. *Above left:* at eight weeks; *above right:* at 13 weeks; and *left:* 19 weeks of gestation. Scans show cephalic pole of the fetus (cf), choroid plexus (CP), lateral ventricle (LV).

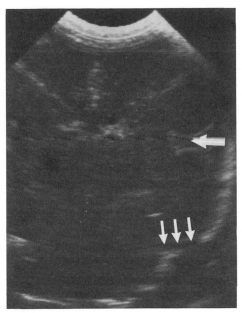

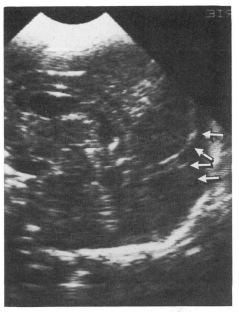

Fig. 2.32. Coronal scan through the middle cranial fossa in a 27-week gestation infant showing normal widening of the Sylvian fissure *(large arrow)* and subarachnoid space *(small arrows)*.

Fig. 2.33. Sagittal scan showing prominence of subarachnoid space and parieto-occipital sulcus *(arrows)* in a 28-week gestation infant.

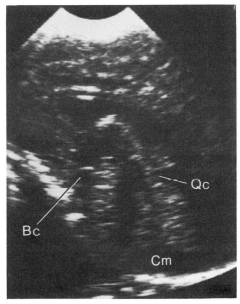

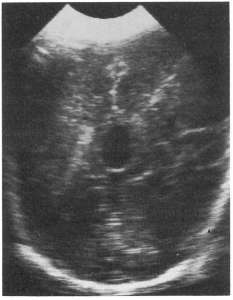

Fig. 2.34. Sagittal scan showing prominence of the quadrigeminal cistern (Qc), basal cistern (Bc) and cisterna magna (Cm).

Fig. 2.35. Coronal scan of posterior cranial fossa showing a prominent echo-free cavum vergae.

the insula by the 40th week, and gives the characteristic 'Y' shape on ultrasound examination (Fig. 2.21). Progression of brain development is evident by the increase in number and depth of sulci appearing in the parenchyma. They become more convoluted and give off many ramifications.

The ventricular system

These are relatively large structures up to the 18th to 20th week, and then reduce proportionately in size. Prominent lateral ventricles may be normally found until the 32nd week. Enlargement of the subarachnoid spaces and prominence of the cisterns are also normally present. The normal ultrasound appearance of the CSF spaces between 28 and 32 weeks' gestation includes an echo-free region located between the brain surface and the skull on coronal and sagittal sections (Fig. 2.33). This represents the normal subarachnoid space. In addition there is prominence of the quadrigeminal cistern, basal cistern and cisterna magna (Fig. 2.34). There is great variability in the size of the subarachnoid space and cisterns at this age.

Several authors have used CT to investigate intra- and extraventricular subarachnoid spaces in children (Ment *et al.* 1981, Kleinmann *et al.* 1983). The subarachnoid spaces were found to be both larger and more variable in size before the age of two years, and to be quite uniform thereafter (Kleinmann *et al.* 1983). To our knowledge, no systematic measurement of the subarachnoid spaces in the premature infant has been evaluated by means of ultrasound.

Cavum septi pellucidi and vergae

These cavities develop in the line of previous fusion of the cerebral hemispheres as a secondary cleavage when the fibres of the corpus callosum cross the midline (Fig. 2.35). They do not communicate with either the subarachnoid or ventricular spaces (Rakic and Yakovlev 1968). These cavities are almost always present in premature infants (Larroche and Baudey 1961). The cavum septi pellucidi closes completely by two months of life (Shaw and Alvord 1969). In rare cases the cavum may enlarge and obliterate the lateral ventricles or foramen of Monro, with subsequent hydrocephalus (Dandy 1931). It is important to recognise the cavum septi pellucidi and to distinguish it from the third ventricle on ultrasound examination. In premature infants it may be surprisingly large. Farrugia and Babcock (1981), in their study of 102 infants, found that the width of the cavum septi pellucidi ranged from 2mm to 10mm, and that the height could be as much as 12mm.

REFERENCES

Babcock, D. S., Han, B. K. (1981) 'The accuracy of high resolution real-time ultrasonography of the head in infancy.' *Radiology*, **139**, 665-676.
—— —— Lequesne, G. W. (1980) 'B-mode gray scale ultrasound of the head in the newborn and young infant.' *American Journal of Roentgenology*, **134**, 457-468.
Couture, A., Cadier, L. (1983) *Echographie Cérébrale par Voie Trans-Fontanellaire*. Paris: Vigot.
Cremin, B. J., Chilton, S. J., Peacock, W. J. (1983) 'Anatomical landmarks in anterior fontanelle ultrasonography.' *British Journal of Radiology*, **56**, 517-526.
Dandy, W. E. (1931) 'Congenital cerebral cysts of the cavum septi pellucidi (fifth ventricle) and cavum vergae (sixth ventricle).' *Archives of Neurology and Psychiatry*, **25**, 44-46.

Farrugia, S., Babcock, D. S. (1981) 'The cavum septi pellucidi: its appearance and incidence with cranial ultrasonography in infancy.' *Radiology*, **139**, 147-150.

Fiske, C. E., Filly, R. A., Callen, P. W. (1981) 'The normal choroid plexus: ultrasonographic appearance of the neonatal head.' *Radiology*, **141**, 467-471.

Goodwin, L., Quisling, R. G. (1983) 'The neonatal cisterna magna: ultrasonic evaluation.' *Radiology*, **149**, 691-695.

Grant, E. G., Schellinger, D., Borts, F. T., McCullough, D. C., Friedmann, G. R., Sivasubramanian, K. N., Smith, Y. (1980) 'Real-time sonography of the neonatal and infant head.' *American Journal of Neuroradiology*, **1**, 487-492.

Johnson, M. L., Mack, L. A., Rumack, C. M., Frost, M., Rashbaum, C. (1979) 'B-mode echoencephalography in the normal and high risk infant.' *American Journal of Roentgenology*, **133**, 375 381.

Kleinmann, P. K., Zito, J. L., Davidson, R. I., Raptopoulos, V. (1983) 'The subarachnoid spaces in children: normal variations in size.' *Radiology*, **147**, 455-457.

Kossoff, G., Garrett, W. J., Radavanovich, G. (1974) 'Ultrasonic atlas of normal brain of infant.' *Ultrasound in Medicine and Biology*, **1**, 259-266.

Larroche, J. C., Baudey, J. (1961) 'Cavum septi pellucidi, cavum vergae, cavum veli interpositi: cavités de la ligne médiane. Etude anatomique et pneumoencephalographique dans la période néonatale.' *Biologia Neonatorum*, **3**, 193-236.

Levene, M. I., Wigglesworth, J. S., Dubowitz, V. (1981) 'Cerebral structure and intraventricular haemorrhage in the neonate: a real-time ultrasound study.' *Archives of Disease in Childhood*, **56**, 416-424.

Ment, L R., Duncan, C. C., Geehr, R. (1981) 'Benign enlargement of the subarachnoid spaces in the infant.' *Journal of Neurosurgery*, **54**, 504-508.

Pigadas, A., Thompson, J. R., Grube, G. L. (1981) 'Normal infant brain anatomy: correlated real-time sonograms and brain specimens.' *American Journal of Roentgenology*, **137**, 815-820.

Rakic, P., Yakovlev, P. I. (1968) 'The development of corpus callosum and cavum septi in man.' *Journal of Comparative Neurology*, **132**, 45-72.

Shaw, C. M., Alvord, C. E. (1969) 'Cava septi pellucidi and vergae. Their normal and pathological states.' *Brain*, **92**, 213-223.

Shuman, W. P., Rogers, J. V., Mack, L. A., Alvord, E. C., Christie, D. P. (1981) 'Real-time sonographic sector scanning of the neonatal cranium: technique and normal anatomy.' *American Journal of Roentgenology*, **137**, 821-828.

3
INTRACRANIAL HAEMORRHAGE

Intracranial haemorrhage is recognised to be a complication of traumatic birth or prematurity. It is more likely to occur within the first 24 hours of life than at any other time, and is now a common cause of death in the premature infant and an important cause of neurodevelopmental handicap in survivors. Until recently, the frequency of intracranial bleeding has been deduced from autopsy data. Craig (1938) found that subdural haemorrhages accounted for half of fatal intracranial haemorrhages and intraventricular haemorrhage was found in only 17 per cent of infants at post-mortem examination. With improvements in obstetric care, subdural haematoma is rarely seen at post-mortem; but intraventricular haemorrhage now accounts for the majority of bleeds found at autopsy, and is common in surviving premature infants. In view of the importance of accurate diagnosis of intraventricular haemorrhage, it is discussed at length in Chapter 4.

The detection rate of various types of intracranial haemorrhage by ultrasound is variable, and it must be stated that sonography may not be the investigation of choice in the diagnosis of all types of haemorrhage. In this chapter we will discuss the value of ultrasound in detecting different types of intracranial haemorrhage, and provide examples of these abnormalities.

Ccphalhaematoma

Cephalhaematoma is not really an intracranial haemorrhage, and usually provides little difficulty in clinical diagnosis. It is due to subperiosteal bleeding over the outer surface of the calvarium and is usually associated with perinatal trauma or forceps delivery. The periosteum confines the cephalhaematoma between cranial sutures, and only crosses the midline in the rare occipital variety. Occasionally confusion between occipital cephalhaematoma and encephalocele may occur. Under these circumstances, ultrasound delineates the blood between the periosteum and overlying skull. The periosteum and skull produce sharp linear echoes, and cephalhaematoma between these structures appears echo-free (Fig. 3.1). By contrast with encephalocele, a skull defect should be detected (Fig. 3.2).

Subdural

This type of haemorrhage is no longer a common condition in the neonate. It is associated with birth trauma, rapid delivery or generalised bleeding disorders. It occurs as a result of tearing of a dural fold, most commonly the tentorium or falx and sometimes rupture of the superficial cerebral bridging veins may occur. Breech delivery, particularly in the preterm infant, may be associated with occipital diastasis, and bleeding originates from venous sinuses as the dura is torn.

The diagnosis of subdural haemorrhage by ultrasound is cited in the literature (Haber *et al.* 1980, Babcock and Han 1981, Slovis and Kuhns 1981, Loxton *et al.*

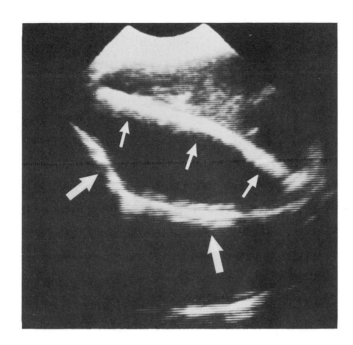

Fig. 3.1. Cephalhaematoma. Transducer is placed on scalp overlying a large parietal swelling. Skull *(larger arrows)* is separated from periosteum *(small arrows)* by echo-free thrombus. There is no skull defect.

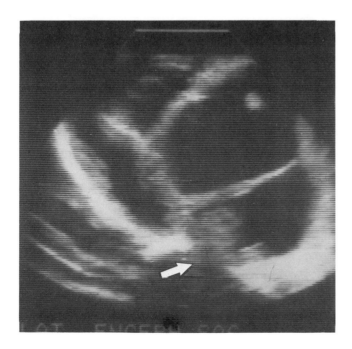

Fig. 3.2. Encephalocele. Transducer has been placed over midline occipital sac. Contents contain cystic and dysplastic neural elements. Echoes from cerebral tissue can be seen penetrating through a skull defect *(arrow)*.

35

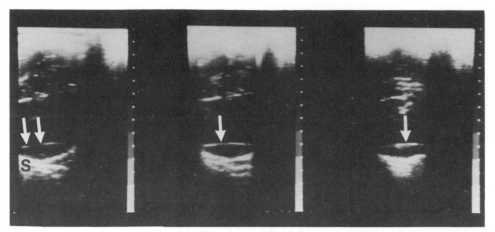

Fig. 3.3. Small subdural haemorrhage. Three axial sections through temporoparietal bone showing opposite table of skull (S) and dura *(arrowed)*. The subdural was confirmed by CT scanning.

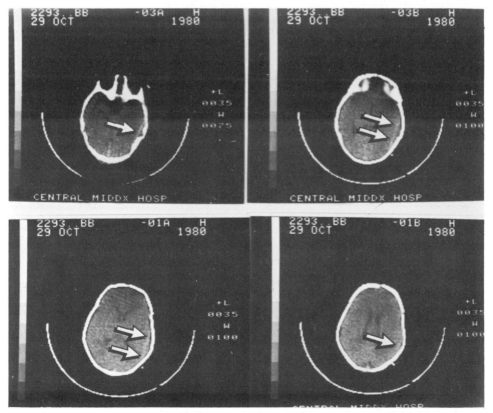

Fig. 3.4. Small subdural haemorrhage. Computerised tomography confirms small subdural collection *(arrowed)* in the same infant illustrated in Figure 3.3.

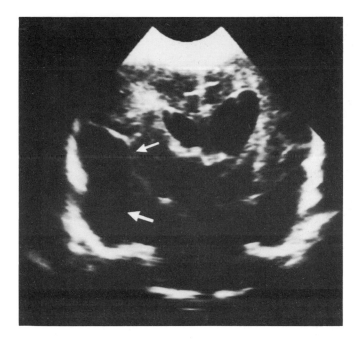

Fig. 3.5. Subdural haemorrhage. Coronal scan from a 29-week gestation infant. An echo-free collection lying in parietal region on left side *(arrowed)*.

1982), but diagnosis depends on the site of the haemorrhage and its size. Convexity haemorrhages (Morgan *et al.* 1983) are easier to detect than those related to the tentorium or due to occipital diastasis. Figures 3.3 and 3.4 show an example of a small convexity subdural detected on axial scanning, which was subsequently confirmed by CT scanning. An axial scan with either linear or sector imaging transducers is probably the best way to pick up a small subdural haemorrhage in this position. Larger collections are often seen on coronal scans, as is shown in Figure 3.5. If a subdural is suspected, care should be taken in viewing the near-field structures; an acoustic coupler or water-path device aids the diagnosis (Slovis and Kuhns 1981, Loxton *et al.* 1982).

It is neither possible confidently to diagnose subdural haemorrhage by ultrasound nor refute its presence. Subarachnoid haemorrhage (see below) and external hydrocephalus (Chapter 11) may give very similar appearances, and as mentioned elsewhere, haemorrhage in the region of the posterior fossa may be easily missed.

Subarachnoid

Subarachnoid haemorrhage (SAH) may be due to blood tracking through the ventricular system from, for example, an intraventricular haemorrhage, or may be primarily due to bleeding from small vessels within the subarachnoid space. Both types of haemorrhage are common. Primary SAH is often seen at autopsy and blood-stained cerebro-spinal fluid (CSF) is frequently obtained at lumbar puncture. Subarachnoid haemorrhage is generally a benign condition, and large bleeds are

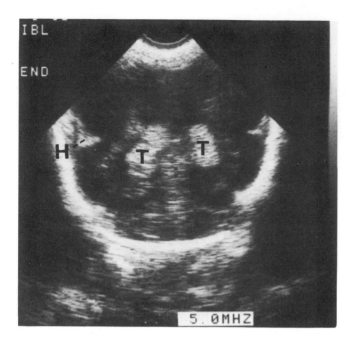

Fig. 3.6. Subarachnoid haemorrhage. Coronal scan showing intraventricular thrombus (T) and echoes in the Sylvian fissure (H) corresponding to thrombus tracking through ventricular system into the subarachnoid space. (Courtesy of Dr. Michael Bilicki.)

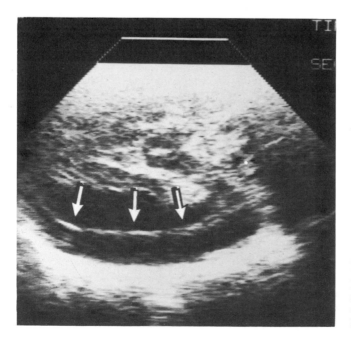

Fig. 3.7. Subarachnoid haemorrhage. Axial scan through temporoparietal bone showing opposite table of skull (thick echo) and arachnoid displaced from skull by thrombus *(arrows)*. This infant had developed a large intraventricular haemorrhage a day before this scan was performed.

38

less common. Symptoms are rare unless cerebral compression occurs associated with a large convexity haemorrhage.

Very few reports exist on the ultrasound detection of SAH, and generally this diagnosis is thought to be extremely unreliable as many false negatives will occur. Quisling *et al.* (1983) suggested that subarachnoid haemorrhage could be detected if widening of the Sylvian fissure or insular sulcus was seen, but correctly diagnosed only one of nine cases by ultrasound compared with CT diagnosis. Babcock *et al.* (1982) stated that a prominent subarachnoid space was commonly seen on early ultrasound scans, but this correlated poorly with the presence of actual SAH over the cerebrum as seen at autopsy. Normally in the very premature infant a prominent subarachnoid space is seen and this should not be confused with the presence of a haemorrhage (Chapter 2). Mack *et al.* (1981) did not detect SAH by ultrasound in any of nine cases in which haemorrhage was subsequently proven at autopsy. In view of these reports it is surprising that Lebed *et al.* (1982), using a linear array machine, claimed to detect SAH in 98 per cent of cases proved by CT scan, and there was only one false positive out of 36 cases with negative CT scans. However, they failed to define the ultrasound appearances of this condition!

The problem with the sonographic diagnosis of SAH is the close proximity of the subarachnoid space to the bone echo. It is extremely unlikely that small volumes of blood will be detected, but it is possible that thrombus within the Sylvian fissure may be recognised. In addition we believe it is almost impossible to distinguish between subarachnoid and subdural haemorrhage.

We have occasionally seen SAH on ultrasound scanning. Figure 3.6 shows the scan of an infant with bilateral intraventricular thrombus, and echoes can be clearly seen in the Sylvian fissure representing thrombus that has tracked through the ventricular system. Another infant with a large intraventricular haemorrhage developed an obvious collection of blood, presumably in the subarachnoid space, seen best on axial views, and causing marked shift of the midline (Fig. 3.7). This mass effect resolved within five days. Coronal scans will detect major SAH particularly if cerebral compression occurs. Figure 3.8 shows an example of massive subarachnoid blood confirmed at autopsy (Fig. 3.9). In conclusion, ultrasound will detect large SAH, but is generally unreliable in view of the large number of false negatives.

Parenchymal

The commonest site of origin for intraparenchymal haemorrhage is extension from a periventricular bleed (Chapter 4). Spontaneous intraparenchymal bleeds are considerably less common but may occur. Diagnosis should not be difficult, as the haemorrhage is seen as strongly echogenic areas within the low echodensity cerebrum. Spontaneous haemorrhage may be due to a generalised bleeding disorder, an angiomatous malformation, trauma or prenatal infection.

Figure 3.10 illustrates massive bilateral spontaneous intraparenchymal haemorrhages in a term infant born with thrombocytopenia. These eventually resolved, to leave large bilateral porencephalic cysts (Fig. 3.11). Another infant showed bilateral parenchymal echoes mainly in the frontal lobe (Fig. 3.12) and at

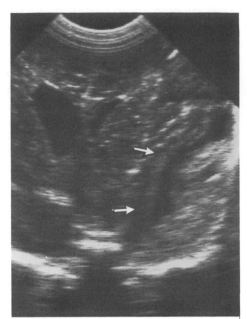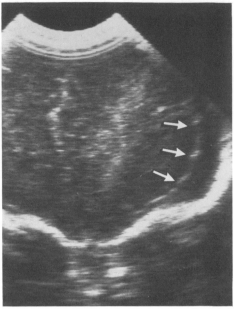

Fig. 3.8. Massive subarachnoid haemorrhage. Thrombus is seen compressing temporoparietal lobe *(above left)* and extending forward *(above right)* into the anterior cranial fossa *(arrows)*. There is a marked midline shift and secondary ventricular dilatation.

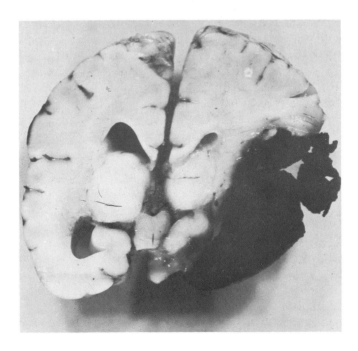

Fig. 3.9. Post-mortem specimen from infant shown in Figure 3.8. There is a large subarachnoid thrombus with considerable parenchymal destruction.

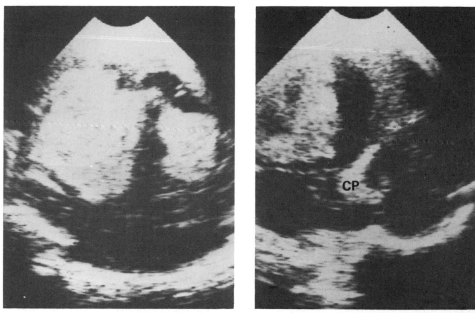

Fig. 3.10. Intraparenchymal haemorrhage. Dense echoes are seen in both occipital poles on coronal view *(above left)*. On parasagittal scan *(right)* the haemorrhage is seen separate from choroid plexus (CP) and there is some liquefaction around the thrombus (scan shows posterior to left). This infant was born with severe thrombocytopenia.

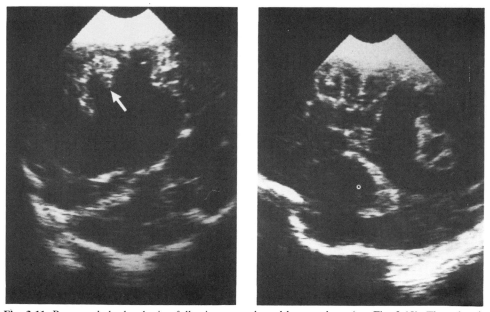

Fig. 3.11. Porencephaly developing following parenchymal haemorrhage (see Fig. 3.10). Thrombus is still visible in left hemisphere *(arrowed)* with some deviation of the midline *(left)*. On parasagittal scans *(right)* extensive porencephaly is seen.

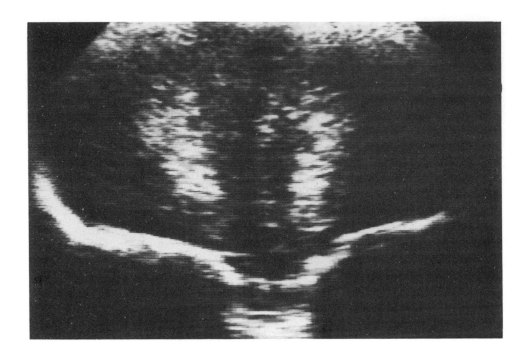

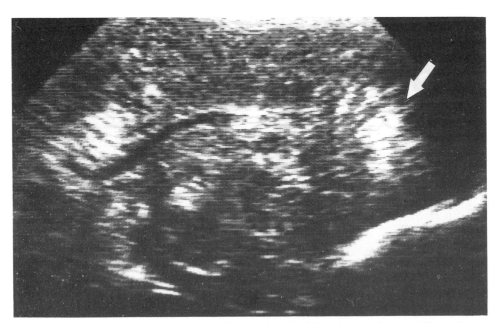

Fig. 3.12. Intraparenchymal haemorrhages. Coronal view *(top)* into the anterior cranial fossa showing bilateral echogenic areas. On parasagittal scan *(bottom)* there were corresponding echoes in the frontal pole *(arrowed,* scan shows posterior to left). See text for details.

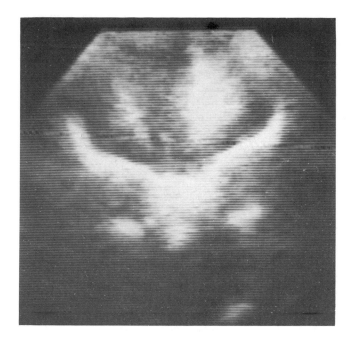

Fig. 3.13. Unilateral parenchymal haemorrhage. This was due to extension of an intraventricular haemorrhage.

autopsy this was seen to be due to multiple petechial haemorrhages probably related to prenatal infection. This may be unilateral (Fig. 3.13).

In order to avoid misdiagnosis, other causes of intraparenchymal echodensity must be considered. These include tumour, infarction, lipoma and vascular abnormalities (these are discussed in detail elsewhere). Slovis and Kuhns (1981) describe an infant with a markedly echogenic parenchymal lesion which was subsequently shown to be a racemose haemangioma.

Thalamic

This type of lesion is very uncommon. Grant *et al.* (1981) describe one case in a term infant in whom complete resolution occurred. In the full-term infants the haemorrhage appears to be primary and the infants present with convulsions (Fig. 3.14). In premature infants the haemorrhage may originate from a germinal matrix bleed, but this is a rare occurrence (Fig. 3.15).

Choroid plexus

Intraventricular bleeding may result from a choroid plexus haemorrhage, but little is known of the frequency and pathogenesis of this condition. Friede (1975) found choroid plexus haemorrhage in only 7 per cent of autopsy specimens, but Reeder *et al.* (1982*a*) diagnosed this type of lesion to be the bleeding site in 10 of the 17 (59 per cent) very low-birthweight babies with intracranial haemorrhage. It is thought that choroid plexus haemorrhage occurs more commonly in infants beyond 36 weeks, and the blood often remains fluid within the ventricles (Pape and

43

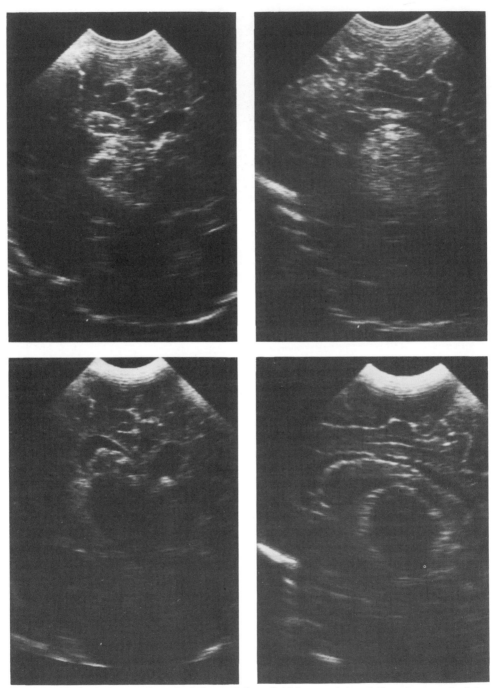

Fig. 3.14. Thalamic haemorrhage in full-term infant. Initial coronal *(top left)* and parasagittal *(top right)* scans show echodensity in region of left thalamus and lateral ventricle. 10 days later there had been marked reduction in echoes within thalamus *(bottom left and right)*.

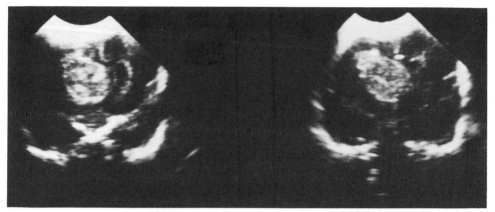

Fig. 3.15. Intrathalamic haemorrhage in a 26-week gestation infant. Coronal views showing extension of intraventricular haemorrhage into the left thalamus. Note deviation in the midline structures.

Wigglesworth 1979).

The ultrasound diagnosis of choroid plexus haemorrhage has been reported occasionally (Sauerbrei *et al.* 1981, Partridge *et al.* 1983), but Reeder *et al.* (1982*a*) have carefully defined the ultrasound appearances of this condition in infants of 1500g and below. Haemorrhage was diagnosed when the choroid plexus appeared enlarged, asymmetrical or irregular in outline. The presence of occipital horn dilatation on the side of the lesion strengthened the diagnosis. Absence of subependymal haemorrhage was also required before haemorrhage of the choroid plexus could be confidently diagnosed. In order to quantify the size of a normal choroid plexus, serial measurements were made; these ranged from 5 to 12mm (mean 7.9mm). In those thought to have haemorrhage, the range was 8 to 19mm (mean 12.2mm). They considered a choroid plexus diameter of 12mm or more to be suggestive of haemorrhage.

We have seen choroid plexus haemorrhage not infrequently in both term and premature infants. The features of this condition are much as described by Reeder *et al.* (1982*a*). Irregularity and increase in size of the choroid plexus is a prerequisite, and thrombus adherent to the choroid filling the temporal pole may be seen (Figs. 3.16 and 3.17). It is likely that minor degrees of choroid plexus bleeding will be overlooked on ultrasound examinations.

Intracerebellar
Cerebellar haemorrhage is now well recognised and may affect both term and immature infants. Intracerebellar haemorrhage usually arises either within the cerebellar cortex or, less commonly, in the subependymal layer of the roof of the fourth ventricle (Pape and Wigglesworth 1979). Venous infarction into the cerebellum may be associated with a tight-fitting face-mask (Pape *et al.* 1976), or

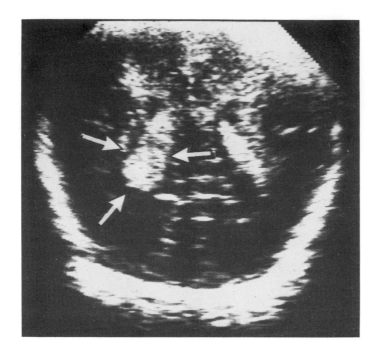

Fig. 3.16. Choroid plexus haemorrhage. Coronal view showing an enlarged pear-shaped choroid on the left *(arrowed)*. This represents thrombus adherent to it, and contrasts with the normal choroid on the other side.

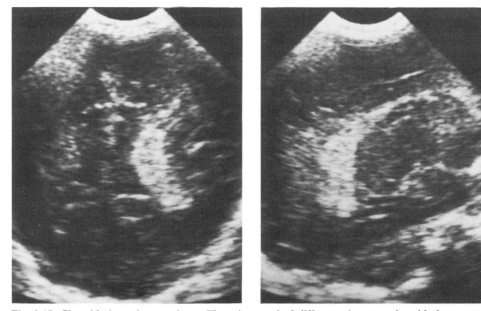

Fig. 3.17. Choroid plexus haemorrhage. There is a marked difference between choroid plexus on the right compared to the left side *(left)*. On parasagittal view *(right)* the choroid is enlarged and fills the trigone.

generalised disorders of coagulation. The incidence of this condition in autopsy data varies from 7 to 12 per cent of very low-birthweight infants (Martin *et al.* 1976, Grunnet and Shields 1976). Diagnosis of posterior fossa haemorrhage by CT is reliable, but resolution of intracerebellar haemorrhage from subdural bleeding is considerably more difficult (Scotti *et al.* 1981). The incidence of cerebellar haemorrhage in the newborn as diagnosed by CT is in the order of 1 per cent (Scotti *et al.* 1981).

Ultrasound diagnosis of massive intracerebellar haemorrhage is now well described in the preterm infant, and in all cases was associated with periventricular haemorrhage (Foy *et al.* 1982, Reeder *et al.* 1982b, Perlman *et al.* 1983). Normally the cerebellum on ultrasound scanning is a pear-shaped structure which appears relatively echodense compared with adjacent cerebral tissue. The sonographic appearance of intracerebellar haemorrhage is a markedly echogenic irregular region in the posterior fossa, best seen to the right or left of the midline. The density of echoes corresponding to haemorrhage is considerably greater than that of the normal cerebellum.

It must be stressed that neither CT nor ultrasound reliably detects intracerebellar haemorrhage, and confusion with tentorial subdural haemorrhage may occur. Large lesions may be detected sonographically, but all too often they will be missed.

REFERENCES

Babcock, D. S., Han, B. K. (1981) 'The accuracy of high resolution, real-time ultrasonography of the head in infancy.' *Radiology,* **139,** 665-676.
—— Bove, K. E., Han, B. K. (1982) 'Intracranial hemorrhage in premature infants: sonographic-pathologic correlation.' *American Journal of Neuroradiology,* **3,** 309-317.
Craig, W. S. (1938) 'Intracranial haemorrhage in the new-born.' *Archives of Disease in Childhood,* **13,** 89-124.
Foy, P., Dubbins, P. A., Waldroup, L., Graziani, L., Goldberg, B. B., Berry, R. (1982) 'Ultrasound demonstration of cerebellar haemorrhage in a neonate.' *Journal of Clinical Ultrasound,* **10,** 196-198.
Friede, R. L. (1975) *Developmental Neuropathology.* Vienna: Springer.
Grant, E. G., Borts, F., Schellinger, D., McCullough, D. L., Smith, Y. (1981) 'Cerebral intraparenchymal haemorrhage in neonates: sonographic appearance.' *American Journal of Neuroradiology,* **2,** 129-132.
Grunnet, M. L., Shields, W. D. (1976) 'Cerebellar haemorrhage in the premature infant.' *Journal of Pediatrics,* **88,** 605-608.
Haber, K., Wachter, R. D., Christenson, P. C., Vaucher, Y., Sahn, D. J., Smith, J. R. (1980) 'Ultrasonic evaluation of intracranial pathology in infants: a new technique.' *Radiology,* **134,** 173-178.
Lebed, M. R., Schifrin, B. S., Waffran, F., Hohler, C. W., Afriat, C. T. (1982) 'Real-time B scanning in the diagnosis of neonatal intracranial hemorrhage.' *American Journal of Obstetrics and Gynecology,* **142,** 851-861.
Loxton, A. J., Schulman, A., Grové, H. (1982) 'Subdural fluid in infants diagnosed using the water-bath technique in ultrasonography.' *South African Medical Journal,* **61,** 858.
Mack, L. A., Wright, K., Hirsch, J. H. (1981) 'Intracranial hemorrhage in premature infants: accuracy of sonographic evaluation.' *American Journal of Roentgenology,* **137,** 245-250.
Martin, R., Roessmann, U., Fanaroff, A. (1976) 'Massive intracerebellar hemorrhage in low birth weight infants.' *Journal of Pediatrics,* **89,** 290-293.
Pape, K. E., Armstrong, D. L., Fitzhardinge, P. M. (1976) 'Central nervous system pathology

associated with mask ventilation in the very low birth weight infant: a new etiology for intracerebellar hemorrhages.' *Pediatrics,* **58,** 473-483.

—— Wigglesworth, J. S. (1979) *Haemorrhage, Ischaemia and the Neonatal Brain. Clinics in Developmental Medicine No. 69/70.* London: SIMP with Heinemann; Philadelphia: Lippincott.

Partridge, J. C., Babcock, D. S., Steichen, J. J., Han, B. K. (1983) 'Optimal timing for diagnostic cranial ultrasound in low birth weight infants: detection of intracranial hemorrhage and ventricular dilatation.' *Journal of Pediatrics,* **102,** 281-287.

Perlmann, J. M., Nelson, J. S., McAlister, W. H., Volpe, J. J. (1983) 'Intracerebellar haemorrhage in a premature newborn: diagnosis by real-time ultrasound and correlation with autopsy findings.' *Pediatrics,* **71,** 159-162.

Quisling, R. G., Reeder, J. D., Setzer, E. S., Kaude, J. V. (1983) 'Temporal comparative analysis of computed tomography with ultrasound for intracranial hemorrhage in premature infants.' *Neuroradiology,* **24,** 205-211.

Reeder, J. D., Kaude, J. V., Setzer, E. S. (1982*a*) 'Choroid plexus hemorrhage in premature neonates. Recognition by sonography.' *American Journal of Neuroradiology,* **3,** 619-622.

—— Setzer, E. S., Kaude, J. V. (1982*b*) 'Ultrasonographic detection of perinatal intracerebellar hemorrhage.' *Pediatrics,* **70,** 385-386.

Sauerbrei, E. E., Digney, M., Harrison, P. B., Cooperberg, P. L. (1981) 'Ultrasonic evaluation of neonatal intracranial hemorrhage and its complications.' *Radiology,* **139,** 677-685.

Scotti, G., Flodmark, O., Harwood-Nash, D. C., Humphries, R. P. (1981) 'Posterior fossa hemorrhages in the newborn.' *Journal of Computer Assisted Tomography,* **5,** 68-72.

Slovis, T. L., Kuhns, L. R. (1981) 'Real-time sonography of the brain through the anterior fontanelle.' *American Journal of Roentgenology,* **136,** 277-286.

4
PERIVENTRICULAR HAEMORRHAGE

Aetiology, frequency and timing

Neonatal periventricular haemorrhage (PVH) is the commonest form of intracranial pathology to be recognised by real time ultrasound, and its pathogenesis and aetiology will be discussed briefly here. The term PVH refers to a spectrum from isolated subependymal haemorrhage to intraventricular rupture and finally parenchymal extension (Pape and Wigglesworth 1979). Subependymal haemorrhage (SEH) refers to haemorrhage arising within the subependymal plate (also called the germinal matrix) located in the region of the head of the caudate nucleus. The subependymal plate produces glial cells which migrate during the midtrimester to the cerebral parenchyma and ganglia, and with increasing gestational age gradual involution of this area occurs. The subependymal plate is most active between 24 and 34 weeks' gestation, this being the time when haemorrhage is most likely to occur. In the full-term infant, the subependymal plate has almost entirely disappeared. It is supplied by a rich matrix of poorly supported fragile capillaries, and it is rupture of these vessels that initiates PVH. Haemorrhage may remain confined to the subependymal plate adjacent to the caudate nucleus, but frequently ruptures upwards into the body of the lateral ventricle, hence the term intraventricular haemorrhage (IVH). In about 20 per cent of cases, further extension may occur mediolaterally through the roof of the lateral ventricle into the cerebral parenchyma.

Periventricular haemorrhage is very occasionally seen in both stillborn infants and full-term surviving infants. As it occurs due to subependymal plate rupture, it is a condition of prematurity. Approximately 30 per cent of infants born before 34 weeks' gestational age develop PVH, and about 50 per cent of those born at 30 weeks of gestation or below (approximately equivalent to 1500g) sustain this lesion. Most haemorrhages have occurred by 72 hours after birth and almost all by seven days of age. Late haemorrhages occurring in the second or third week have been reported but are rare. The onset of the haemorrhage within the first 72 hours varies between different neonatal intensive care units. Most commonly PVH occurs with roughly equal frequency in the first, second and third 24-hour periods, but very early onset (before six hours from birth) occurs in some centres.

Diagnosis

The first reports of ultrasound detection of IVH appeared in the late 1970s (Heimburger *et al.* 1978, Johnson *et al.* 1979, Pape *et al.* 1979), and modifications and improvements to these methods rapidly occurred. Pape *et al.* (1979) initially reported the diagnosis of PVH by a linear array real-time machine imaging in an axial plane through the temporo-parietal region (Fig. 4.1). Johnson and colleagues detected haemorrhages, using both a static B-mode machine and a linear array

49

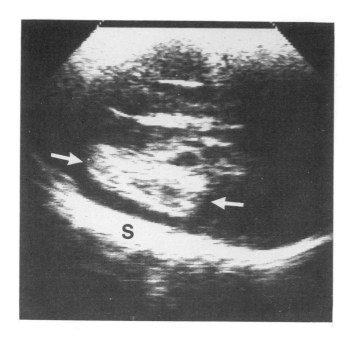

Fig. 4.1. Axial scan showing parenchymal extension of a periventricular haemorrhage. The haemorrhage *(arrowed)* lies medial to the skull echo (S).

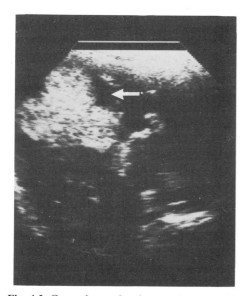 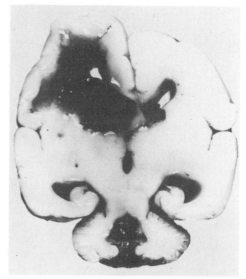

Fig. 4.2. Coronal scan showing massive parenchymal extension of a periventricular haemorrhage *(left)*. The actual haemorrhage is shown on the right for comparison. There is some liquefaction of thrombus within the parenchyma and this is seen as an echo-free area on the scan *(arrow)*.

real-time scanner, but this method had the obvious disadvantage of transporting the baby to the scanning device—a procedure likely to further compromise an infant requiring intensive care. Trans-fontanelle scanning with a real-time machine, as originally suggested by Cooke (1979) and Allan *et al.* (1980), rapidly became accepted as the best technique for neonatal brain scanning, and made the detection, staging and follow-up of haemorrhage reliable (Fig. 4.2).

As discussed in the section on normal appearances (Chapter 2) the brain can be visualised in three planes—coronal, sagittal and axial—and haemorrhage can also be studied in these planes. Haemorrhages vary considerably in size and position and depending on whether intraparenchymal extension has occurred.

Small SEH usually develops adjacent to the head of the caudate nucleus at the level of, or just anterior to, the foramen of Monro and appears as discrete echo-dense areas. In its most minor degree, little if any distortion of the ventricular outline occurs; and a homogenous echogenic area is seen at the inferolateral margin of the lateral ventricle (Figs. 4.3 to 4.5). In these cases it is important to confirm this area on sagittal scans before diagnosing PVH. Mild degrees of PVH commonly appear as subependymal echoes with mild ventricular dilatation, which is usually asymmetrical and transient (Fig. 4.6). This may be due to distension of the ventricle by liquid unclotted blood which produces no echoes. Bilateral SEH is usually slightly asymmetrical, and if completely symmetrical, careful examination in sagittal plane must be made before confident diagnosis of PVH is made.

If thrombus forms in the ventricles, intraventricular echoes will be seen (Fig. 4.5). These may fill a small part of the ventricular system or form a complete cast of one or both lateral ventricles. Intraventricular thrombus may be confined to the occipital poles of the lateral ventricles. Not uncommonly, echogenic thrombi are seen in the third ventricle and temporal poles of the lateral ventricles. Thrombus in the fourth ventricle is rarely identified. Some infants show the appearance of bright linear echoes in the region of the floor of the lateral ventricle (Fig. 4.7) which results from sound-waves striking the ependyma perpendicularly with complete reflection. Care must be taken to ensure that these normal specular echoes are not confused with a small SEH.

Parenchymal involvement is most common in the temporo-parietal and occipital regions. These haemorrhages are usually wedge-shaped in coronal section, and it is often difficult to distinguish between SEH, ventricular thrombus and parenchymal haemorrhage. Complete examination of the brain is necessary to ascertain the maximal size of PVH, because considerable extension may occur into the occipital pole without involvement of more anterior parenchymal tissue (Figs. 4.8 and 4.9). It is rare to find extension of an IVH into the parenchyma anterior to the frontal pole of the lateral ventricle.

Progressive extension of a PVH may occur in a small proportion of infants, and frequent scanning will best detect this progression. Figure 4.10 shows examples of progressive extension from a small SEH to massive intraparenchymal lesions. The frequency with which small haemorrhages slowly progress to large ones is not clear. Levene and de Vries (1984) found this to occur in 13 per cent of cases of PVH whereas Partridge *et al.* (1983) report extension to occur in up to 43 per cent of

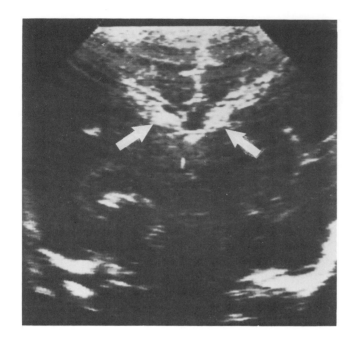

Fig. 4.3. Small bilateral periventricular haemorrhages seen as discrete echogenic regions in the region of the subependymal plate *(arrows)*.

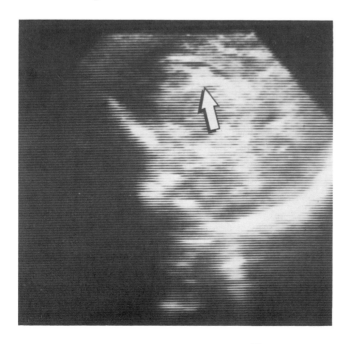

Fig. 4.4. Small subependymal haemorrhage seen on parasagittal scan as an echodense lesion in the thalamo-caudate notch *(arrowed)*.

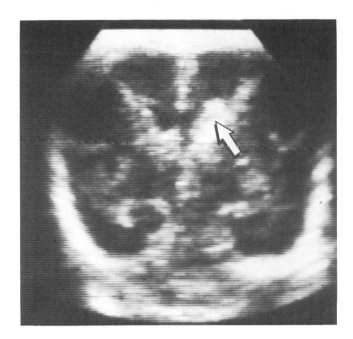

Fig. 4.5. Right-sided intraventricular haemorrhage. An echodense area is shown filling the right lateral ventricle *(arrowed)*.

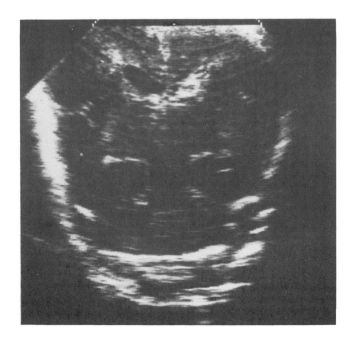

Fig. 4.6. Contralateral ventricular dilatation with right-sided haemorrhage. The ventricular dilatation resolved within 10 days.

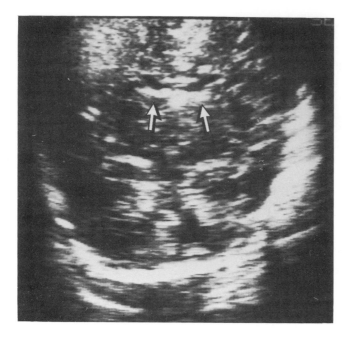

Fig. 4.7. Normal scan showing linear echoes *(arrows)* resulting from sound waves striking the floor of lateral ventricle (see text). It is important not to confuse this appearance with small subependymal haemorrhages.

cases. The extension continued to occur up to 21 days of age.

Resolution of haemorrhage follows a similar pattern whether it be intracerebral or intraventricular. Over the period of two to three weeks, reduction in the density of echoes occurs at the centre of the previous uniformly echogenic haemorrhage. This continues until only a thin echogenic rim remains. Within the ventricles, thrombi may become detached and gradually reduce in echodensity until eventually they disappear completely.

Accuracy of diagnosis

Surprisingly, there are few good studies on the accuracy of ultrasound in the diagnosis of PVH. Correlation has been attempted in two ways; ultrasound compared to autopsy, and ultrasound against computerised tomography (CT). Errors may occur in both types of comparison. Although autopsy must be the standard against which all imaging techniques should be compared, an interval between the last scan and death may have been associated with a new haemorrhage or extension of an old one. Ultrasound and CT depend on quite different physical properties in order to generate an image, and the detection rates of haemorrhage may not be the same when the two techniques are compared.

From autopsy data the correlation between ultrasound and post-mortem findings show agreement in 78 to 90 per cent of these cases (see Table 4.1). These studies compare different types of ultrasound modalities (usually linear array or static B-mode), and few have carefully analysed the accuracy of modern real-time sector scanners. Major degrees of haemorrhage were usually accurately detected

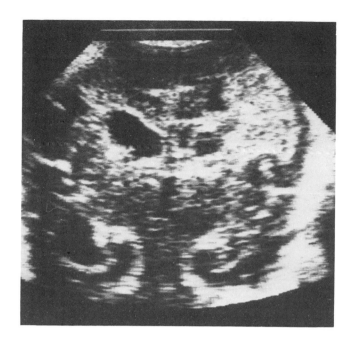

Fig. 4.8. Intraparenchymal haemorrhage arising from a right-sided periventricular bleed.

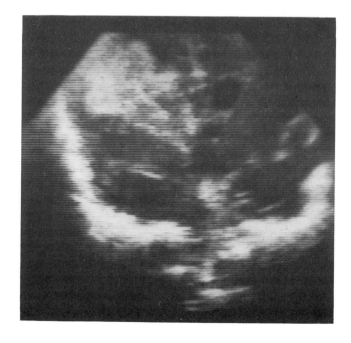

Fig. 4.9. Massive parenchymal extension into left hemisphere.

TABLE 4.1

Correlation between ultrasound and autopsy diagnosis of PVH. Static refers to a static B-mode scanner and sector to a real-time sector scanner

	Type of scanner	Agreement between autopsy and US	Autopsy positive US negative	Autopsy negative US positive
Babcock *et al.* (1982)	Static/sector	22 of 25 (88%)	5	1
Levene *et al.* (1982)	Linear/sector	26 of 29 (90%)	0	3
Thorburn *et al.* (1982)	Linear	34 of 38 (89%)	3	1
Pape *et al.* (1983)*	Linear	117 of 150 (78%)	20	13
	Static	95 of 120 (88%)	13	12

*Each hemisphere was considered separately for SEH, IVH and intraparenchymal haemorrhage. 25 patients were studied with linear array and 20 with static scanning and the figures reflect various haemorrhages in different areas of the brain.

TABLE 4.2

Grading systems for PVH used or adapted for use with ultrasound brain scanning

Papille *et al.* 1978	Gd. I	Isolated SEH
	Gd. II	Rupture into ventricle, but no dilatation
	Gd. III	Rupture into ventricle with dilatation
	Gd. IV	IVH with parenchymal extension
Lazzara *et al.* 1980	Mild	SEH ± ventricular blood filling ≤25% of the ventricles
	Moderate	IVH with blood filling 25–50% of the ventricles
	Severe	IVH with blood filling ≥50% of the ventricles
Levene *et al.* 1982	Gd. I	Haemorrhage in region of germinal matrix with no extension
	Gd. II	Downward extension or thrombus in lateral ventricle
	Gd. III	Parenchymal extension
Shankaran *et al.* 1982	Mild	SEH ± small amount of blood in normal sized ventricles
	Moderate	Intermediate amount of blood in enlarged ventricles
	Severe	IVH filling entire lateral ventricle forming a cast ± parenchymal haemorrhage

TABLE 4.3

A modification of the grading system suggested by Levene and de Crespigny (1983) which describes the extent of haemorrhage and ventricular dilatation separately. For follow-up purposes the maximum grade of haemorrhage should be recorded

Haemorrhage	0 – No haemorrhage
	1 – Localised haemorrhage ≤1cm in its largest measurement
	2 – Haemorrhage >1cm in its largest measurement but not extending beyond the atrium of the lateral ventricle
	3 – Blood clot forming a cast of the lateral ventricle and extending beyond the atrium
	4 – Intraparenchymal haemorrhage
Ventricular dilatation	0 – No dilatation
	1 – Transient dilatation
	2 – Persistent but stable dilatation
	3 – Progressive ventricular dilatation requiring treatment
	4 – Persistent asymmetrical ventricular dilatation

56

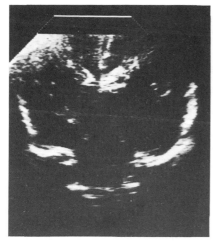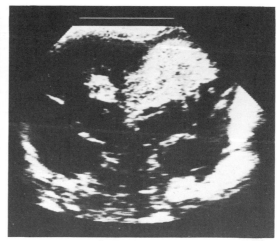

Fig. 4.10. Extension of haemorrhage. *Two coronal scans from same infant taken at 18 (left) and 43 hours (right) from birth. In first scan there is small periventricular haemorrhage mainly on right. 25 hours later, massive right-sided parenchymal extension had occurred. (Reproduced by courtesy of the editors of the Archives of Disease in Childhood.)*

and presented few problems in diagnosis. In three of these four studies, ultrasound tended to under-diagnose haemorrhage. Those lesions overlooked tended to be small and confined to the subependymal plate. Correlation between ultrasound and CT varied between 50 and 100 per cent agreement (Silverboard *et al.* 1980, Johnson *et al.* 1981, Thorburn *et al.* 1982, Quisling *et al.* 1983). The reasons for poor correlation depended on the presence or absence of intraventricular blood and the age of the haemorrhage when CT scanning was performed. With CT, intracranial blood may become isodense with brain within five to seven days from the haemorrhage, and thus will not be seen. When CT itself is compared to autopsy, correlation has been reported to be as high as 91 per cent (Flodmark *et al.* 1980*a*).

Failure of ultrasound to diagnose some cases of PVH accurately can be considered in a number of different ways. These include size of the lesion, anatomical localisation of the haemorrhage, detection of intraventricular blood, and echodensities due to non-haemorrhagic causes. The minimal size of haemorrhage that can be visualised by ultrasound has rarely been carefully considered. Pape *et al.* (1983) found that lesions of 5mm or below were poorly demonstrated by both linear array (5MHZ transducer) and a static B-mode scanner (5MHZ short focus probe). It is possible that with modern high quality sector scanners fitted with a 7MHZ transducer, the detection rate of small lesions may improve.

The normal choroid plexus is the most likely structure to be misdiagnosed as haemorrhage. The normal choroid plexus has been discussed in Chapter 2. It is an intensely echogenic structure, broad posteriorly and closely related to the pulvinar of the thalamus, tapering anteriorly to be no longer visible at the level of the foramen of Monro. Its anterior-most extension, however, is somewhat variable, and it is easily confused with small SEH. Subependymal haemorrhage is usually seen

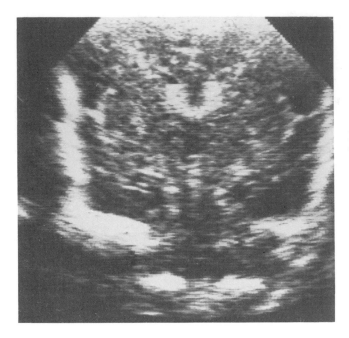

Fig. 4.11. Mistaken diagnosis of periventricular haemorrhage. Bilateral echogenic lesions were first noted by day 10 in a 30-week infant. They showed no subsequent change until death at three weeks of age. Autopsy did not detect haemorrhage, but echoes corresponded in anatomical position to fornices. The medial position of these echoes contrast with the slightly more lateral position of subependymal plate haemorrhages.

anterior to, and separate from, the choroid echo. Irregularity at the anterior portion of the choroid echo should be evident if haemorrhage is present. Bilateral symmetrical areas of apparent SEH must be carefully inspected and distinguished from normal choroid plexus before confident diagnosis of haemorrhage can be made.

Figure 4.11 shows a mistaken diagnosis of bilateral SEH. This appearance was not present at birth, developed at 10 days of age and then showed no further change. Autopsy revealed no haemorrhage and the position of the echoes corresponded with the fornices. In retrospect these echoes are unusually symmetrical and too medial to be SEH.

Thrombus within the lateral ventricles produces obvious echoes, but it is uncertain whether or not ultrasound detects unclotted blood in the ventricles. Mack *et al.* (1981) correctly diagnosed SEH by ultrasound, but failed to detect small amounts of intraventricular blood in five out of 12 cases. Silverboard and his colleagues (1980) maintained that fresh blood in the ventricles may not be detected by ultrasound within five days from the onset of haemorrhage. Babcock *et al.* (1982) make the point that enlargement of the lateral ventricles by anechoic fluid indicates IVH but the blood has been diluted by cerebrospinal fluid. This has also been our experience. Figure 4.6 shows asymmetrical dilatation of the lateral ventricles associated with echoes in the region of the subependymal plate. We believe that blood within the ventricles does not produce echoes when in the fluid phase. Furthermore, correlation between ultrasound-diagnosed IVH and autopsy data is considerably worse (67 per cent) than correlation with either intracerebral haemorrhage (92 per cent) or SEH (76 per cent) (Pape *et al.* 1983). Conversely Bejar *et al.* (1980) claimed to detect liquid blood both *in vivo* and *in vitro* down to a haematocrit of 2 per cent. Confirmation for this has not yet been forthcoming.

Echodensity within the brain may occur due to other forms of pathology including oedema, calcification, lipomata, intravascular air and tumour and are discussed elsewhere. Intraparenchymal echoes are usually due to extension of IVH into the cerebral white matter but infarction, both venous and arterial, may also cause an identical appearance on ultrasound scans. Other imaging techniques may be necessary to resolve these questions and will be discussed further in Chapter 13.

Grading of PVH

Unfortunately there is no generally accepted method for grading the extent of PVH, and to date there have been at least eight different systems described in the literature (Papille *et al.* 1978, Krishnamoorthy *et al.* 1979, Lazzara *et al.* 1980, Mantovani *et al.* 1980, Hutchson and Fleischer 1981, Levene *et al.* 1982, Shankaran *et al.* 1982, Levene and de Crespigny 1983). Four of these were originally devised for use in CT scanning (Papille *et al.* 1978, Krishnamoorthy *et al.* 1979, Lazzara *et al.* 1980, Mantovani *et al.* 1980). The CT grading system of Papille *et al.* has been adopted for use in ultrasound scanning, and is described in Table 4.2. As discussed above, it is unlikely that ultrasound accurately distinguishes ruptured from unruptured SEH; thus distinction between Papille Grade I and II cannot reliably be made with ultrasound. The CT grading system of Lazzara *et al.* has also been used for sonography (Silverboard *et al.* 1980) and does not make a distinction between ruptured and unruptured SEH. The ultrasound grading systems of Shankaran *et al.* and Levene *et al.* also do not attempt to make this distinction. These systems are also described in Table 4.2, and we consider them to be more appropriate to ultrasonography than the system of Papille and colleagues.

Most grading systems include the size of the lateral ventricles (Papille *et al.* 1978, Krishnamoorthy *et al.* 1979, Lazzara *et al.* 1980, Mantovani *et al.* 1980, Hutchson and Fleischer 1981, Shankaran *et al.* 1982, Levene and de Crespigny 1983) but Flodmark *et al.* (1980*b*) questioned the validity of this. They studied the relation between the ventricular size, degree of IVH and postnatal age. Those infants examined after two days not only had larger ventricles, but showed increasingly severe enlargement for each progressive grade of IVH. Their work suggests that after two days of age, the ventricular size is as much related to the postnatal age as the extent of haemorrhage. For these reasons they felt that neither the amount of ventricular blood nor the size of the ventricles were a good index to use in grading PVH. From their data, there seem to be good reasons why PVH and ventricular size should be graded separately. Recently Levene and de Crespigny (1983) described a grading system for PVH which does just that (Table 4.3). Ventricular dilatation is discussed fully in Chapter 5.

Timing of scans

Almost all periventricular haemorrhages occur within the first week of life and the majority by 72 hours from birth. The risk of PVH is highly correlated with the degree of prematurity; those infants above 34 weeks' gestation are unlikely to develop this condition. A protocol for routine scanning should therefore concentrate on those infants most likely to develop PVH (<34 weeks gestation or <2000g birthweight). In addition to these infants, ill babies with abnormal neurological signs (seizures, apathy, irritability) should be scanned to detect the rare case of PVH that occurs in more mature infants. If routine scanning is undertaken for the diagnosis of PVH then the first scan should be performed by the end of the first week of life. Partridge *et al.* (1983) studied PVH in infants of birthweight 1500g and below, and found 96 per cent of their infants developed haemorrhage by seven days and 100 per cent by day 14. It is unlikely that significant PVH will have resolved by seven days, and we would agree that two scans at seven and 14 days should detect almost all periventricular haemorrhages in at-risk infants.

REFERENCES

Allan, W. C., Roveto, C. A., Sawyer, L. R., Courtney, S. E. (1980) 'Sector scan ultrasound imaging through the anterior fontanelle: its use in diagnosing neonatal periventricular-intraventricular hemorrhage.' *American Journal of Diseases of Children,* **134,** 1028-1031.

Babcock, D. S., Bove, K. E., Han, B. K. (1982) 'Intracranial hemorrhage in premature infants: sonographic-pathologic correlation.' *American Journal of Neuroradiology,* **3,** 309-317.

Bejar, R., Curbelo, V., Coen, R. W., Leopold, J., James, H., Gluck, L. (1980) 'Diagnosis and follow-up of intraventricular and intracerebral hemorrhages by ultrasound studies of infant's brain through the fontanelles and sutures.' *Pediatrics,* **66,** 661-673.

Cooke, R. W. I. (1979) 'Ultrasound examination of neonatal heads.' *Lancet,* **2,** 38. *(Letter).*

Flodmark, O., Becker, L. E., Harwood-Nash, D. C., Fitzhardinge, P. M., Fitz, C. R., Chuang, S. H. (1980a) 'Correlation between computed tomography and autopsy in premature and full term neonates that have suffered perinatal asphyxia.' *Radiology,* **137,** 93-103.

—— Fitz, C. R., Harwood-Nash, D. C. (1980b) 'CT diagnosis and short-term prognosis of intracranial hemorrhage and hypoxic/ischemic brain damage in neonates.' *Journal of Computer Assisted Tomography,* **4,** 775-787.

Heimburger, R., Fry, F., Patrick, J. T., Gardner, G., Gresham, E. (1978) 'Ultrasound brain tomography for infants and young children.' *Perinatology/Neonatology,* **2,** 27-31.

Hutchson, A. A., Fleischer, A. C. (1981) 'A classification of neonatal intracranial hemorrhage.' *New England Journal of Medicine,* **305,** 284.

Johnson, M. L., Mack, L. A., Rumack, C. M., Frost, M., Rashbaum, C. (1979) 'B-mode echoencephalography in the normal and high risk infant.' *American Journal of Roentgenology,* **133,** 375-381.

—— Rumack, C. M., Mannes, E. J., Appareti, K. E. (1981) 'Detection of neonatal intracranial hemorrhage utilising real-time and static ultrasound.' *Journal of Clinical Ultrasound,* **9,** 427-434.

Krishnamoorthy, K. S., Shannon, D. C., DeLong, G. R., Todres, I. D., Davis, K. R. (1979) 'Neurologic sequelae in the survivors of neonatal intraventricular hemorrhage.' *Pediatrics,* **64,** 233-237.

Lazzara, A., Ahmann, P., Dykes, F., Brann, A. W., Schwartz, J. (1980) 'Clinical predictability of intraventricular hemorrhage in preterm infants.' *Pediatrics,* **65,** 30-34.

Levene, M. I., de Crespigny, L. Ch. (1983) 'Classification of intraventricular haemorrhage.' *Lancet,* **1,** 643.

—— de Vries, L. (1984) 'Extension of intraventricular haemorrhage.' *Archives of Disease in Childhood,* **59,** 631-636.

—— Fawer, C.-L., Lamont, R. F. (1982) 'Risk factors in the development of intraventricular haemorrhage in the preterm neonate.' *Archives of Disease in Childhood,* **57,** 410-417.

Mack, L. A., Wright, K., Hirsch, J. H. (1981) 'Intracranial hemorrhage in premature infants: accuracy of sonographic evaluation.' *American Journal of Roentgenology,* **137,** 245-250.

Mantovani, J. F., Pasternak, J. F., Mathew, O. P., Allan, W. C., Mills, M. T., Casper, J., Volpe, J. J. (1980) 'Failure of daily lumbar punctures to prevent the development of hydrocephalus following intraventricular hemorrhage.' *Journal of Pediatrics,* **97,** 278-281.

Pape, K. E., Cusick, G., Houang, M. T. W., Blackwell, R. J., Sherwood, A., Thorburn, R. J., Reynolds, E. O. R. (1979) 'Ultrasound detection of brain damage in preterm infants.' *Lancet,* **2,** 1261-64.

—— Wigglesworth, J. S. (1979) *Haemorrhage, Ischaemia and the Perinatal Brain. Clinics in Developmental Medicine No. 69/70.* London: SIMP with Heinemann: Philadelphia: Lippincott.

—— Bennett-Britton, S., Szymonowicz, W., Martin, D.J., Fitz, C. R., Becker, L. (1983) 'Diagnostic accuracy of neonatal brain imaging: a post-mortem correlation of computed tomography and ultrasound scans.' *Journal of Pediatrics,* **102,** 275-280.

Papille, L. A., Burstein, J., Burstein, R., Koffler, H. (1978) 'Incidence and evolution of subependymal and intraventricular hemorrhage: a study of infants with birth weight less than 1500gm.' *Journal of Pediatrics,* **92,** 529-534.

Partridge, J. C., Babcock, D. S., Steichen, J. J., Han, B. K. (1983) 'Optimal timing for diagnostic cranial ultrasound in low birth-weight infants: detection of intracranial hemorrhage and ventricular dilatation.' *Journal of Pediatrics,* **102,** 281-287.

Quisling, R. G., Reeder, J. D., Setzer, E. S., Kaude, J. V. (1983) 'Temporal comparative analysis of computed tomography with ultrasound for intracranial hemorrhage in premature infants.' *Neuroradiology,* **24,** 205-211.

Shankaran, S., Slovis, T. L., Bedard, M. P., Poland, R. L. (1982) 'Sonographic classification of intracranial hemorrhage. A prognostic indicator of mortality, morbidity, and short-term neurologic outcome.' *Journal of Pediatrics,* **100,** 469-475.

Silverboard, G., Horder, M. H., Ahmann, P. A., Lazzara, A., Schwartz, J. F. (1980) 'Reliability of ultrasound in the diagnosis of intracranial hemorrhage and posthemorrhagic hydrocephalus: comparison with computed tomographic scan.' *Pediatrics,* **66,** 507-514.

Thorburn, R. J., Lipscomb, A. P., Reynolds, E. O. R., Blackwell, R. J., Cusick, G., Shaw, D. G., Smith, J. F. (1982) 'Accuracy of imaging of the brains of newborn infants by linear-array real-time ultrasound.' *Early Human Development,* **6,,** 31-46.

5
SEQUELAE OF PVH

The natural history of PVH is unpredictable, and although complete resolution of the ultrasound appearances occurs in the majority of cases, complications and sequelae of the haemorrhage may develop in a significant proportion of cases. These include ventricular dilatation, porencephaly and cystic degeneration at the site of the original haemorrhage. All of these can be readily detected by ultrasound.

Post-haemorrhagic ventricular dilatation

Some enlargement in size of the lateral ventricles occurs in up to 40 per cent of infants surviving acute PVH, but only a minority (approximately 5 to 10 per cent of those developing PVH) require ventricular shunting for progressive hydrocephalus. Although ventricular dilatation following haemorrhage is common, there is now evidence that it may be associated with an increased risk of adverse neurodevelopmental outcome (Palmer *et al.* 1982). For these reasons, all infants who have sustained PVH should be scanned regularly to detect an increase in ventricular size. Effective treatment and the eventual prognosis may depend on its early recognition. Post-haemorrhagic ventricular dilatation also occurs from other causes of haemorrhage, including subarachnoid bleeds and choroid plexus haemorrhage, but these are considerably less common initiating events than PVH.

As discussed in Chapter 4, acute IVH may commonly cause alteration in size of the lateral ventricles. This is probably due to distension of one or both ventricles by liquid blood. When this occurs it usually produces asymmetric and only mildly dilated ventricles (Fig. 5.1). This is due to obstruction to the flow of cerebrospinal fluid, and should not be confused with the symmetrical ventricular dilatation occurring five days or more after the onset of IVH.

Cerebrospinal fluid (CSF) is produced by the choroid plexus situated in the occipital poles of the lateral ventricle, and is also found in the third and fourth ventricles. The total volume of CSF replaces itself several times a day, and any degree of obstruction to flow will rapidly lead to ventricular dilatation. The CSF formed by the choroid plexus flows through the foramen of Monro into the third ventricle, and then into the fourth ventricle through the aqueduct of Sylvius. Fluid leaves the brain from the fourth ventricle into the subarachnoid space through the foramina of Luschka and Magendie or the central canal of the spinal cord. Absorption of fluid is achieved at the arachnoid granulations over the surface of the brain. Blockage of the arachnoid granulations is the commonest site of obstruction following haemorrhage, and is termed 'communicating hydrocephalus'. The next most likely site of blockage is at the base of the skull as the CSF leaves the fourth ventricle; this is termed 'non-communicating obstruction' or 'intraventricular obstructive hydrocephalus' (IVOH).

The terminology relating to ventricular dilatation is confusing. Hydrocephalus

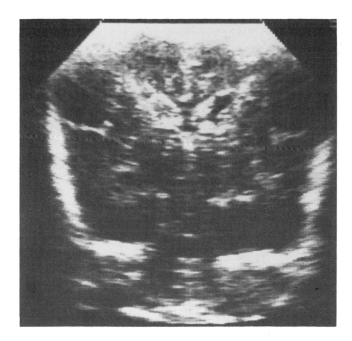

Fig. 5.1. Univentricular dilatation due to echo-free liquid blood within right ventricular cavity. Thrombus (strongly echogenic) is seen within left ventricle.

is a descriptive term used for many years to denote a *clinical* appearance, including rapid head-growth, dilated scalp veins, sunsetting sign of the eyes with perhaps lethargy and vomiting. With the introduction of newer imaging techniques, it became apparent that ventricular dilatation preceded abnormal head-growth by days or weeks (Volpe *et al.* 1977). It is not yet clear from prospective ultrasound examinations of the brain exactly when the term 'post-haemorrhagic hydrocephalus' should be used. We believe it is best to continue to use it only as a clinical description. Ventriculomegaly has also been used to describe ventricular dilatation not progressing to hydrocephalus (Allan *et al.* 1982), and others use the term 'arrested hydrocephalus' to refer to a similar appearance. When ventricular

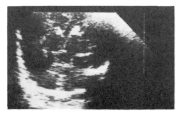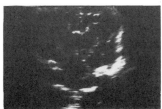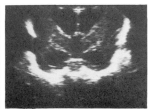

Fig. 5.2. Progressive ventricular dilatation. Three coronal scans from 32-week gestation infant. At three days of age, echoes corresponding to small bilateral intraventricular haemorrhage is seen with normal ventricular size *(left)*. At eight days of age, both lateral ventricles are dilated *(centre)*; by three weeks of age, massive dilatation of the lateral and third ventricle is apparent *(right)*. This infant required ventricular shunt.

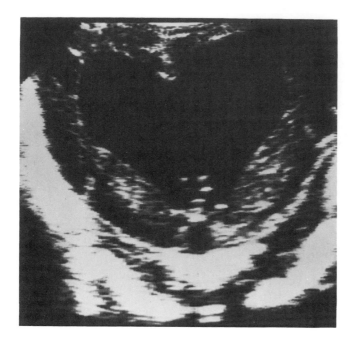

Fig. 5.3. Massive dilatation of
lateral ventricles. The lateral
and third ventricles contain
echo-free cerebrospinal fluid.
Note the small paraventricular
cysts in left hemisphere.

dilatation occurs following haemorrhage it is impossible to know whether it will
become progressive or not. We suggest that the term 'post-haemorrhagic
ventricular dilatation' be used to describe an increase in size of the ventricles
following PVH. At discharge from the neonatal unit it may be possible to state
whether this was transient, persistent or progressive (Levene and Starte 1981).

Figures 5.2 to 5.5 show examples of post-haemorrhagic ventricular dilatation.
Any degree of intraventricular blood may be associated with this condition, but
infants most at risk are those who sustain large ventricular bleeds and in whom the
thrombus forms a cast of the lateral ventricle. Although no figures are available,
our impression is that the majority of infants with this type of haemorrhage go on to
develop significant ventriculomegaly, and may require surgical intervention.

Ventricular dilatation is usually first seen as crescentic enlargement lateral to
the echogenic intraventricular thrombus. This may progress at a variable rate over
days or weeks (Fig. 5.2). Ventricular dilatation following haemorrhage may
become massive, and other pathology (such as cystic degeneration) may be seen to
accompany it (Fig. 5.3). Ventricular enlargement is usually first seen in the
occipital horns of the lateral ventricles, but there is considerable variation in the
size of this part of the ventricular system in normal babies. Occipital dilatation
progressively develops to include all parts of the lateral ventricles. As ventricular
dilatation develops, the walls of the ventricular system often appear to become
more prominent. This may be due to periventricular oedema from exudation of
fluid through the ependyma, or ependymal gliosis secondary to the pressure of
intraventricular blood.

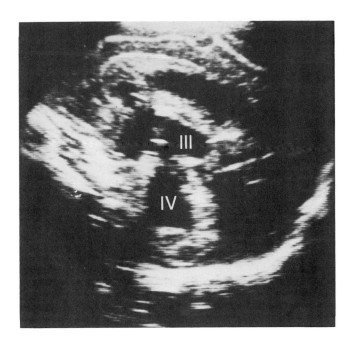

Fig. 5.4. Dilatation of third (III) and fourth (IV) ventricles. Note interthalamic connexus (echogenic structure) within third ventricle.

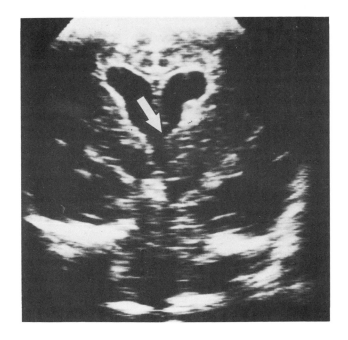

Fig. 5.5. Dilated foramen of Monro (*arrow*) seen connecting the two dilated lateral ventricles.

It is usually possible to see dilatation of the third and fourth ventricles at the time the lateral ventricles dilate (Fig. 5.4). The foramen of Monro is particularly obvious at this stage (Fig. 5.5). Once the lateral ventricles are massively dilated, the third and fourth ventricles may become difficult to detect. At present there seems to be no consistently reliable ultrasound method to distinguish communicating from non-communicating obstruction.

A relatively common sequel to ventricular dilatation is detachment of intraventricular thrombi from the ependyma. Figures 5.6 to 5.8 show stages in this process. Clots floating freely within dilated lateral ventricles are occasionally seen (Fawer and Levene 1982). Gentle turning of the infant's head to different positions causes the thrombus to float gradually to a dependent position (Fig. 5.8). There is a theoretical risk that the thrombus may float into a position which causes acute obstruction to CSF flow, but this does not appear to occur in practice. The thrombi usually disappear within two to four weeks after detachment. The echogenic thrombus gradually becomes less dense, initially in its centre, and later becomes fainter before becoming completely iso-echoic with CSF.

Variable asymmetry in the size of dilated ventricles has also been reported with the larger ventricle on the dependent side. The dependent ventricle may become considerably more dilated than the upper one within four hours of head-turning (Fawer and Levene 1982). This interesting observation has little practical significance. Persistent asymmetrical dilatation is also seen frequently in infants who have had a stormy neonatal course. This may not be due to obstruction, but may be associated with cerebral atrophy. This condition is further discussed in Chapter 10.

In order to detect post-haemorrhagic ventricular dilatation, scans must be performed regularly following haemorrhage. We would suggest a regimen of weekly scans following the diagnosis of PVH. These should continue until the ventricular size is stable for a period of at least several weeks.

Three patterns of ventricular dilatation have been recognised: transient, persistent and progressive ventricular enlargement (Levene and Starte 1981). Following haemorrhage some infants exhibit a temporary increase in size of lateral ventricles. This reaches a maximum by about two to four weeks, and may spontaneously resolve *without* treatment. Persistent dilatation may occur for months or years following initial detection, but is non-progressive and remains in the same proportion to the size of the infant's head. Progressive enlargement leads to clinical hydrocephalus and may require surgical or drug treatment.

Measurement systems
In order to detect ventricular dilatation, a normal range for ventricular size must be established. There is no consensus, and a number of different methods exist. The width of the ventricles may be expressed as a ratio of the total width of the cranium, the ventricles may be measured directly, or an estimate of CSF volume attempted. These methods will now be considered separately.

Lateral ventricular size has been measured for many years by a variety of techniques. Dandy (1918) was the first to publish data on ventricular size visualised

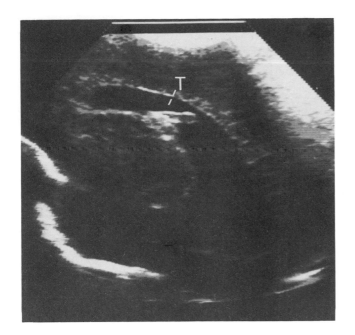

Fig. 5.6. Thrombus (T) lying within body of the lateral ventricle, but still partially attached to floor of lateral ventricle.

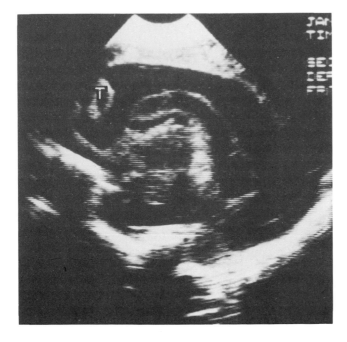

Fig. 5.7. Partially adherent thrombus seen on parasagittal scan. There is a round echogenic thrombus (T) completely detached and freely mobile at anterior pole of lateral ventricle.

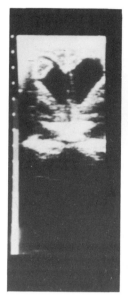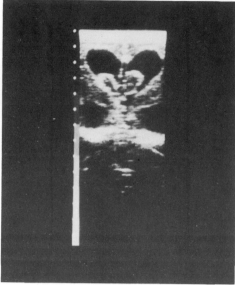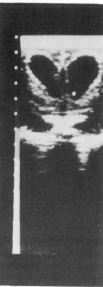

Fig. 5.8. Floating thrombi. Three linear array coronal scans with infant's head lying in different positions. Thrombi are freely mobile. *Left:* when head is lying laterally on left side, visible thrombus floats to left. *Centre:* when head is prone, thrombi lie close to foramen of Monro; and with infant on his back *(right)*, they float out of vision to occipital pole. (Reproduced by courtesy of the editors of the Archives of Disease in Childhood.)

by introducing air into the lateral ventricle. Direct measurement of the size of the lateral ventricles at air ventriculography was not considered reliable, and a ratio was adopted relating the transverse diameter of the anterior horns of the lateral ventricle to the maximum internal diameter of the skull—the Evans ratio (Evans 1942). The introduction of computerised tomography permitted less invasive measurement of the ventricles, but little data is available for the range of ventricular size in normal infants.

Pellici *et al.* (1979) found 95 normal CT scans in a group of 400 patients ranging from newborn to 15 years, in whom the ventricular size could be measured. This was expressed as a ratio of the distance between the heads of the caudate nuclei and the diameter of the cerebral hemispheres. This ratio did not change with age.

Using A-mode ultrasound equipment, various estimates of the ratio of ventricular width to skull diameter in normal newborn infants have been made (Brahme and Tragardh 1969, Dill 1971). Valkeakari (1973), using both A-mode and B-mode techniques, made actual measurements of the width of the body of a single ventricle in normal infants during the first week of life. He found consistent agreement between the two ultrasound display systems. With the widespread use of static B-mode scanning, more precise visualisation of ventricular structure and size could be made. Lombroso *et al.* (1968) used this method and stated that there was little increase in the transverse diameter of the lateral ventricles from one day to one year of age. Two studies using grey-scale B-mode scanning devices reported

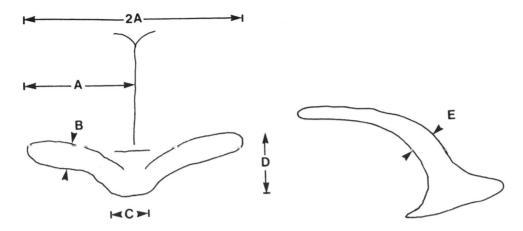

Fig. 5.9. Measurements of lateral ventricular system in coronal planes *(left)* and parasagittal planes *(right).* A—Levene 1981, Sauerbrei *et al.* 1981, Lipscomb *et al.* 1983. 2A—Skolnick *et al.* 1979, London *et al.* 1980. B—London *et al.* 1980. Sauerbrei *et al.* 1981. C—London *et al.* 1980. D—Levene and Starte 1981. E—Allan *et al.* 1982, Quisling *et al.* 1983.

relative size of the ventricular system (Johnson *et al.* 1979, Morgan *et al.* 1979). Johnson *et al.* expressed a ratio of the mean width of the lateral ventricle to the hemispheric measurement, while Morgan *et al.* determined a lateral ventricular ratio from the maximum width of the body of the lateral ventricle and the biparietal diameter. Using linear array real-time ultrasound, Pape *et al.* (1979) also measured a 'ventricle/brain ratio' as the distance between the midline and the lateral wall of the lateral ventricle, related to the distance between the midline and the linear skull table.

Despite widespread use of various types of ratios, we believe direct measurement of the ventricles to be better. Growth cannot be monitored reliably with a ratio, and abnormalities of both ventricle and cortex may not produce an abnormality when expressed as a ratio. Ideally an actual measurement should be used, as this will provide more information on changes in the size of the normal and abnormal ventricles.

With modern real-time ultrasound scanners, clear visualisation of the lateral ventricles can be obtained and exact anatomical landmarks identified. From these, precise measurements can be made. Skolnick *et al.* (1979) measured the biventricular width of the lateral ventricles from outer wall to outer wall, and derived from that the individual width of each lateral ventricle usually at the frontal horn position (Fig. 5.9). London *et al.* (1980) made four measurements: biventricular at the level of the frontal horns, diagonal width of the frontal horns at the level of the caudate nucleus, intercaudate distance, and biventricular at the body of the lateral ventricles. These are also shown in Figure 5.9. They found a progressive increase in all measurements with advancing maturity of the infants. Levene (1981) measured the ventricular size from midline to the lateral-most point of the lateral ventricle (referred to as the ventricular index—VI) in 273 infants from

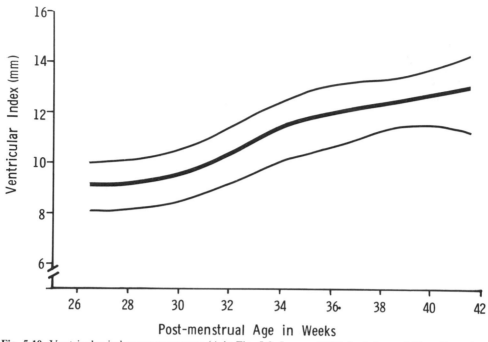

Fig. 5.10. Ventricular index measurements (A in Fig. 5.9. Levene 1981) for infants of 26 to 42 weeks' gestation. Upper and lower lines represent the ±2 standard deviations, and middle line is the mean. (Reproduced by courtesy of the editors of the Archives of Disease in Childhood.)

26 to 42 weeks' gestation. This measurement could be made in either coronal or axial planes. In coronal section the measurement was made at the level of the hippocampal echo, just posterior to the foramen of Monro, and showed little inter-observer error. A centile chart expressing the third, 50th and 97th centiles from 26 to 42 weeks was produced and is shown in Figure 5.10. Recently Lipscomb *et al.* (1983) produced similar data to that of Levene. In addition, the perpendicular measurement from the base of the lateral ventricle to the maximum height in a perpendicular direction was recorded in infants with enlarged ventricles (Levene 1981). Sauerbrei *et al.* (1981), in addition to using a measurement similar to the ventricular index, recorded the depth of the lateral ventricle, defined as the widest measurement taken perpendicular to the longest axis of the lateral ventricle on coronal section (Fig. 5.9). Allan *et al.* (1982) chose to measure ventricular diameter of the lateral ventricle in sagittal plane. This was done at the mid-body near the atrium of the ventricle (Fig. 5.9), but they produced no data for normal babies. A similar measurement was suggested by Quisling *et al.* (1983). Some authors have compared these various ultrasound measurements with CT imaging and found good correlation (Skolnick *et al.* 1979, London *et al.* 1980, Sauerbrei *et al.* 1981).

The variety of different systems for measurement probably results from the irregular manner that the ventricles enlarge when dilatation occurs. As mentioned earlier, the occipital poles tend to enlarge before the body of the lateral ventricles,

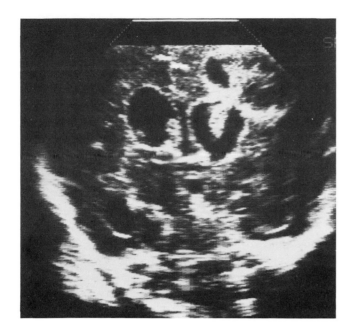

Fig. 5.11. Early porencephalic cyst arising from a right-sided parenchymal haemorrhage. There is an echo-free area surrounding thrombus which is seen present within both cyst and dilated ventricular cavity.

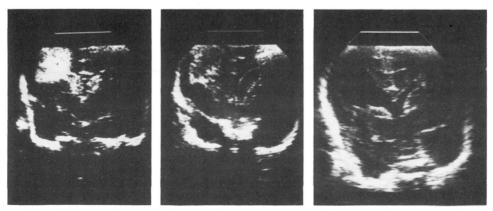

Fig. 5.12. Serial scans showing development of a porencephalic cyst. The scan on the left was made at 48 hours of age in a 28-week gestation infant. There is extensive left-sided parenchymal haemorrhage. Three weeks later *(centre scan)* there has been a considerable reduction in density of parenchymal echoes corresponding to organisation of the thrombus. By eight weeks from birth *(right scan)* there is an echo-free cavity directly communicating with lateral ventricle, occupying area of original haemorrhage.

but measurements in this plane are impracticable in view of the wide range of normal size and shape of occipital poles. The biventricular diameter is also unreliable because one ventricle may enlarge more rapidly than the other. Data has been accumulated and a chart produced for the ventricular index (Levene 1981), and this appears to be a reliable index of ventricular size. Interestingly, the data of Johnson *et al.* for fetal ventricular size measured on axial section is very similar to Levene's ventricular index over a similar gestational age. When ventricular dilatation occurs, the ventricular index is not very sensitive to the early changes. For this reason we also recommend measurement of the depth of the lateral ventricles (London *et al.* 1980, Sauerbrei *et al.* 1981), which increases as soon as dilatation occurs. In normal infants, the roof and floor of the lateral ventricles are closely opposed, and this measurement cannot be made in the normal state.

So far we have discussed measurement in one or two directions in order to monitor any increase in the size of the ventricles. When ventricular dilatation occurs, there is an increase in volume of CSF, and linear measurements do not reflect this change. Horbar *et al.* (1980*b*) suggested the measurement of lateral ventricular cross-sectional area when dilatation occurred. This was done by planimetry of multiple coronal sections, but this more exact method is not practical for routine clinical use.

To date there is no data for the measurement of the cerebral ventricular system other than the lateral ventricles. The third ventricle is not usually visualised on coronal scan when normal, and it must be dilated to be clearly seen. The fourth ventricle is difficult to measure due to its complicated shape and poor delineation on ultrasound.

Porencephaly

Porencephaly refers to an intraparenchymal cyst, but it is a non-specific term, and may result from a number of different pathophysiological mechanisms. This condition is discussed in more detail in Chapter 7. One cause of paraventricular porencephalic cyst formation is resolution of intraparenchymal haemorrhage, and it occurs in about one half to two thirds of infants surviving intraparenchymal haemorrhage. The evolution of porencephalic cysts following PVH has a characteristic course which has been well described in the literature (Pasternak *et al.* 1980, Donn and Bowerman 1982, Grant *et al.* 1982). Figures 5.11 and 5.12 show examples of paraventricular porencephalic cysts and their development from the haemorrhagic stage.

Initially the intraparenchymal haemorrhage is very echogenic, but over two to three weeks the echoes begin to reduce in intensity. Further resolution usually occurs initially around the edge of the haemorrhagic area leaving an echo-free rim. Contraction of the echodense central thrombus continues to occur with encroachment of the echo-free area to leave a definite 'lining' to the developing cyst (Fig. 5.11). Eventually a large echo-free cavity remains which is in direct communication with the lateral ventricle and the mature cyst occupies an area very closely related in size to the original parenchymal haemorrhage (Fig. 5.12). This process usually takes three to eight weeks for complete development.

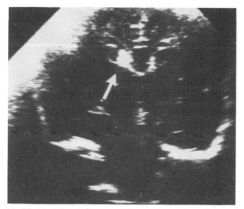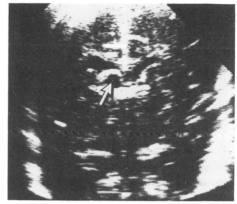

Fig. 5.13. Development of a subependymal pseudocyst. Left-sided periventricular haemorrhage seen at two days of age *(left)*. This was replaced by an echo-free 'subependymal pseudocyst' *(arrow)* by three weeks of age *(right)*.

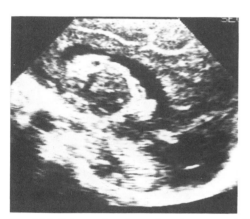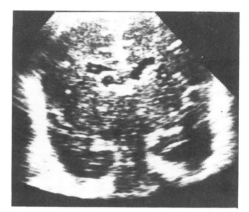

Fig. 5.14. Subependymal pseudocyst on coronal *(left)* and parasagittal *(right)* scans.

Single paraventricular porencephalic cysts must be distinguished from cystic periventricular leukomalacia (Chapter 6). These latter cysts are usually multiple, small and not in obvious communication with the ventricular system. The pathogenesis of the porencephalic cyst is probably due to focal cerebral destruction by the haemorrhage itself, rather than ischaemia or infarction as is the case with cystic periventricular leukomalacia (Pasternak *et al.* 1980).

Subependymal pseudocyst

An echo-free cavity developing at the site of a small subependymal haemorrhage is a relatively common finding on sequential ultrasound scans. Although haemorrhage is the usual cause (Levene 1980), it has been recognised by ultrasound following ventriculitis (Horbar *et al.* 1980*a*). Characteristic examples of this condition are shown in Figures 5.13 and 5.14. The cysts appear by about four weeks after haemorrhage and may eventually disappear completely on sequential ultrasound examinations.

Larroche (1972) reviewed 22 cases seen at post-mortem, and the lesions were usually located in the subependymal germinal matrix at the floor of the lateral ventricle adjacent to the foramen of Monro. This is the usual site in immature infants for periventricular haemorrhages of the germinal matrix origin. The cavity is lined with a thick glial 'felt-work' rather than ependymal epithelium, hence the term pseudocyst. Larroche considered either haemorrhage or infection to be the cause of this lesion, the cyst simply being a marker of previous pathology. The presence of the cyst after SEH appears to confer no additional risk-factor to neuro-developmental outcome.

REFERENCES

Allan, W. C., Holt, P. J., Sawyer, L. R., Tito, A. M., Meade, S. K. (1982) 'Ventricular dilatation after neonatal periventricular-intraventricular hemorrhage.' *American Journal of Diseases of Children,* **136,** 589-593.

Brahme, F., Trägårdh, B. (1969) 'Echoencephalographic estimation of size of the lateral cerebral ventricles in normal children.' *Radiology,* **92,** 60-64.

Dandy, W. E., (1918) 'Ventriculography following injection of air into the cerebral ventricles.' *Annals of Surgery,* **68,** 5-11.

Dill, R. (1971) 'Echoencephalographische normalwerte des Kindlichen ventrikelsystems in den verschiedenen altersgruppen.' *Monatsschrift für Kinderheilkunde, 119,* 496-502.

Donn, S. M., Bowerman, R. A. (1982) 'Neonatal post-hemorrhagic porencephaly. Ultrasonographic features.' *American Journal of Diseases of Children,* **136,** 707-709.

Evans, W. A. (1942) 'An encephalographic ratio for estimating ventricular enlargement and cerebral atrophy.' *Archives of Neurology and Psychiatry,* **47,** 931-937.

Fawer, C.-L., Levene, M. I. (1982) 'Elusive blood clots and fluctuating ventricular dilatation after neonatal intraventricular haemorrhage'. *Archives of Disease in Childhood,* **57,** 158-160.

Grant, E. G., Kerner, M., Schellinger, D., Borts, F. T., McCullough, D. C., Smith, Y., Sivasubramanian, K. N., Davitt, M. K. (1982) 'Evolution of porencephalic cysts from intra-parenchymal haemorrhage in neonates: sonographic evidence.' *American Journal of Roentgenology,* **138,** 467-70 (see also: *American Journal of Neuroradiology,* **3,** 47-50).

Horbar, J. D., Philip, A. G. S., Lucey, J. F. (1980*a*) 'Ultrasound scan in neonatal ventriculitis.' *Lancet,* **1,** 976.

—— Walters, C. L., Philips, A. G. S., Lucey, J. F. (1980*b*) 'Ultrasound detection of changing ventricular size in post-hemorrhagic hydrocephalus.' *Pediatrics,* **66,** 674-678.

Johnson, M. L., Mack, L. A., Rumack, C. M., Frost, M., Rashbaum, C. L. (1979) 'B-mode echoencephalography in the normal and high risk infant.' *American Journal of Roentgenology,* **133,** 375-381.

Larroche, J. C. (1972) 'Sub-ependymal pseudocysts in the newborn.' *Biology of the Neonate,* **21,** 170-183.

Levene, M. I. (1980) 'Diagnosis of lsub-ependymal pseudocysts with cerebral ultrasound.' *Lancet,* **2,** 210-211.

—— (1981) 'Measurement of the growth of the lateral ventricles in preterm infants with real-time ultrasound.' *Archives of Disease in Childhood,* **56,** 900-904.

—— Starte, D. R. (1981) 'A longitudinal study of post-haemorrhagic ventricular dilatation in the newborn.' *Archives of Disease in Childhood,* **58,** 905-910.

Lipscomb, A. P., Thorburn, R. J., Stewart, A. L., Reynolds, E. O. R., Hope, P. L. (1983) 'Early treatment for rapidly progressive post-haemorrhagic hydrocephalus.' *Lancet,* **1,** 1438-1439.

Lombroso, C. T., Erba, G., Yogo, T., Logowitz, N. (1968) 'Two-dimensional ultrasonography: a method to study normal and abnormal ventricles.' *Pediatrics,* **42,** 157-174.

London, D. A., Carroll, B. A., Enzmann, D. R. (1980) 'Sonography of ventricular size and germinal matrix hemorrhage in premature infants.' *American Journal of Neuroradiology,* **1,** 295-300.

Morgan, C. L., Trought, W. S., Rothman, S. J., Jiminez, J. P. (1979) 'Comparison of gray-scale ultrasonography and computed tomography in the evaluation of macrocrania in infants.' *Radiology* **132**, 119-123.

Palmer, P., Dubowitz, L. M. S., Levene, M. I., Dubowitz, V. (1982) 'Developmental and neurological progress of preterm infants with intraventricular haemorrhage and ventricular dilatation.' *Archives of Disease in Childhood*, **57**, 748-753.

Pape, K. E., Cusick, G., Houang, M. T. W., Blackwell, R. J., Sherwood, A., Thorburn, R. J., Reynolds, E. O. R. (1979) 'Ultrasound detection of brain damage in preterm infants.' *Lancet*, **2**, 1261-1264.

Pasternak, J. F., Mantovani, J. F., Volpe, T. J. (1980) 'Porencephaly from periventricular intracerebral hemorrhage in a premature infant.' *American Journal of Diseases of Children*, **134**, 673-675.

Pelicci, L. J., Bedrick, A. D., Cruse, R. P., Vanucci, R. C. (1979) 'Frontal ventricular dimensions of the brain in infants and children.' *Archives of Neurology*, **36**, 852-854.

Quisling, R. G., Reeder, J. D., Setzer, E. S., Kaude, J. V. (1983) 'Temporal comparative analysis of computed tomography with ultrasound for intracranial haemorrhage in premature infants.' *Neuroradiology*, **24**, 205-211.

Sauerbrei, E. E., Digney, M., Harrison, P. B., Cooperberg, P. L. (1981) 'Ultrasonic evaluation of neonatal intracranial hemorrhage and its complications.' *Radiology*, **139**, 677-685.

Skolnick, M. L., Rosenbaum, A. E., Matzuk, T., Guthkelch, A. N., Heinz, E. R. (1979) 'Detection of dilated cerebral ventricles in infants: a correlative study between ultrasound and computed tomography.' *Radiology*, **131**, 447-452.

Valkeakari, T. (1973) 'Analysis of serial echoencephalograms in healthy newborn infants during the first week of life.' *Acta Paediatrica Scandinavica*, Suppl. 242, 1-62.

Volpe, J. J., Pasternak, J. F., Allan, W. C. (1977) 'Ventricular dilatation preceding rapid head growth following neonatal intracranial hemorrhage.' *American Journal of Diseases in Children*, **131**, 1212-1215.

6
ISCHAEMIC CEREBRAL LESIONS IN THE PRETERM AND TERM INFANT

Ultrasound has been extensively used in the diagnosis of periventricular haemorrhage and post-haemorrhagic ventricular dilatation. These conditions are the commonest type of intracranial pathology occurring in the premature infant. The rôle of ultrasound in the identification of hypoxic-ischaemic lesions is still controversial, but recently several studies have provided evidence that ultrasound may give valuable information in the diagnosis of these conditions (Hill *et al.* 1982, Couture and Cadier 1983, Fawer *et al.* 1983, Hill *et al.* 1983, Levene *et al.* 1983).

The outcome of hypoxic-ischaemic brain insult depends on three factors: (i) gestational age, (ii) the nature of the insult, and (iii) the timing of the event. The mesencephalon develops first with growth of the basal ganglia, midbrain and brainstem. The blood supply follows the structural development, and up to 28 weeks' gestation there is a predominance of vessels to these central structures. From 32 to 34 weeks, changes in the pattern of the cerebral vasculature occur with disappearance of the germinal matrix together with rapid growth of the cortex and the white matter. There is a striking increase in the vascular requirement to these regions. Cortical vessels proliferate, and by term the cortical arterial supply is well developed (Hambleton and Wigglesworth 1976, Wigglesworth and Pape 1978). Basic forms of hypoxic-ischaemic damage may be understood in terms of anatomical maturation of the nervous system, together with advancing vascular development.

The cerebral lesions found in the fetus and newborn infants represents the endstage in a sequence of pathological processes designated as anoxic, hypoxic, ischaemic and hypoxic-ischaemic (Leech and Alvord 1974, Myers 1975, Volpe 1976), but in practice these aetiological factors are usually mixed. There is mainly an impairment of brain energy production caused by a deprivation of oxygen (Volpe 1981) or reduced cerebral perfusion. Among premature infants birth asphyxia, recurrent apnoea, severe idiopathic respiratory distress syndrome, bradycardia, cardiac arrest and shock are all common causes of cerebral ischaemia, while perinatal asphyxia represents the major insult in term newborns (Brown *et al.* 1974, Ziegler *et al.* 1976). In the premature infant, the cerebral damage is most often in the periventricular white matter. In the more mature brain the cortex, white matter, basal ganglia, cerebellum and brainstem are most vulnerable to these types of insults (Smith *et al.* 1974).

Periventricular leukomalacia
Periventricular leukomalacia (PVL) is an ischaemic lesion which occurs most commonly in premature infants, although it has occasionally been reported in

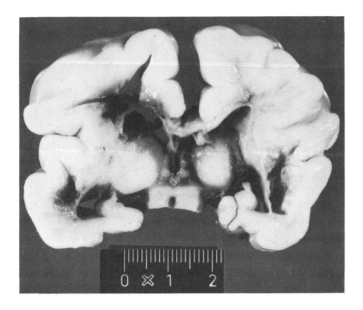

Fig. 6.1. Brain of a 28-week gestation infant dying at two weeks of age, showing intraventricular haemorrhage and extensive periventricular leukomalacia involving right hemisphere and both temporo-occipital regions.

full-term babies (Armstrong and Norman 1974). The lesion was first described by Virchow, and then by Parrot, who recognised these periventricular lesions as 'pale infarcts' (Virchow 1867, Parrot 1873). A comprehensive study of 51 post-mortem specimens was performed by Banker and Larroche (1962). They described for the first time the clinico-pathological condition, and the term 'periventricular leukomalacia' was introduced. Severe perinatal anoxia was identified as the most important aetiological factor. De Reuck *et al.* (1971) and Armstrong and Norman (1974) attributed these lesions to an impairment of perfusion in the terminal distribution of central and cortical arterial supplies or to interarterial 'border zones'. The periventricular white matter adjacent to the external corners of the lateral ventricles have been shown to lie in an arterial 'watershed' region (Pape and Wigglesworth 1979).

Macroscopic and histological changes are characterised by multiple periventricular infarcts affecting the periventricular white matter and sparing the grey matter. The lesions are often bilateral, a few millimetres in diameter and remain separated from the ventricles by a layer of glial tissue. The usual anatomical distribution is in the periventricular white matter adjacent to the anterior region of the frontal horns, the external angle of the lateral ventricles, and the lateral surfaces of the occipital horns (Fig. 6.1) (Friede 1975, Shuman and Selednik 1980).

The earliest microscopic features of PVL correspond to a coagulation necrosis with nuclear pyknosis. The acute lesion is often delineated at its edges by bands of bright red staining, or may sometimes be associated with secondary haemorrhage within the area of necrosis (Armstrong and Norman 1974, Friede 1975). After a few days astrocytic degeneration is seen, microglia proliferates and lipid-laden macrophages accumulate in the necrotic tissue. The lesion becomes well delineated

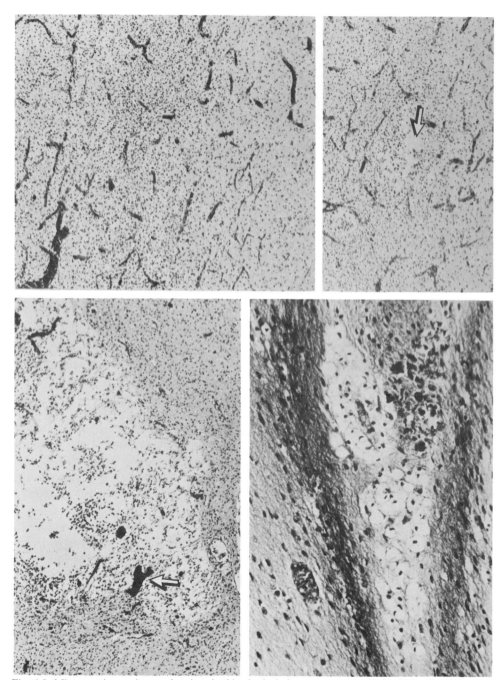

Fig. 6.2. Microscopic specimens showing the histological changes associated with PVL. *Top left:* early lesions with marked vascular congestion. *Top right:* coagulation necrosis and nuclear pyknosis with early cavitation *(arrow)*. *Bottom left:* early mineralisation *(arrow)* with extensive cavitation. *Bottom right:* gliotic stage with lipid-laden macrophages.

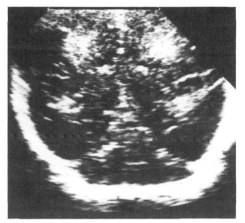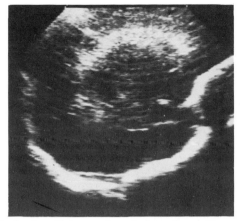

Fig. 6.3. Coronal scan *(left)* and parasagittal *(right)*, showing distinct periventricular echoes with no evidence of periventricular haemorrhage. (Scans show posterior to left.)

by reactive gliosis, and cavitation occurs with formation of cysts of various sizes and shapes. These cavities are surrounded by areas of gliosis. These changes are shown histologically in Figure 6.2.

Most of the published observations of PVL are from post-mortem studies (Banker and Larroche 1962, De Reuck *et al.* 1972, Armstrong and Norman 1974, Shuman and Selednik 1980). The frequency of PVL derived from these studies ranges from 7 to 88 per cent (Banker and Larroche 1962, Leech and Alvord 1974, Shuman and Selednik 1980).

Techniques for identifying this condition in living infants have been very limited. Computerised tomography has been disappointing in the diagnosis of PVL (Di Chiro *et al.* 1978, Estrada *et al.* 1980, Flodmark *et al.* 1980, Hirabayashi *et al.* 1980). Hill *et al.* (1982) reported one case of haemorrhagic PVL in which the diagnosis was made by ultrasound before death, and was subsequently confirmed at autopsy. Two recent studies provide evidence that it is possible to recognise PVL on ultrasound examinations (Fawer *et al.* 1983, Levene *et al.* 1983).

The incidence of this condition based on the ultrasound diagnosis has been reported by Levene *et al.* (1983), who found cystic PVL in 7.5 per cent of very low-birthweight infants. Fawer *et al.* (1983) have shown a slightly higher incidence among premature infants of 34 weeks' gestation and below. Periventricular haemorrhage and PVL frequently co-exist in the same brain (Armstrong and Norman 1974, Shuman and Selednik 1980, Fawer *et al.* 1983, Levene *et al.* 1983), although De Reuck *et al.* (1972) did not find any cases of haemorrhage in their specimens with PVL.

On ultrasound examination, the earliest stage of PVL is characterised by areas of increased echodensity localised to the region of the periventricular white matter, usually in the vicinity of the external angle of the lateral ventricles. These areas have a characteristic triangular shape with the apex pointing towards the ventricle and the base towards the cortex. These ultrasound changes should be apparent in

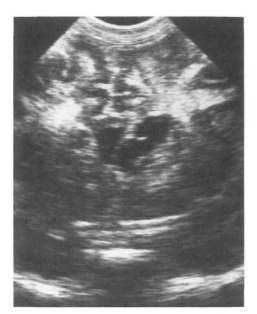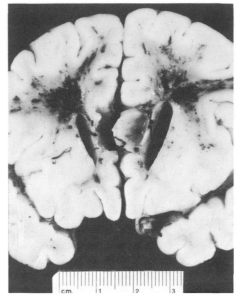

Fig. 6.4. Coronal scan *(left)* and post-mortem specimen *(right)* showing marked periventricular echoes corresponding with region of venous infarction in infant with superior sagittal sinus thrombosis. Thrombosis was not detected by ultrasound.

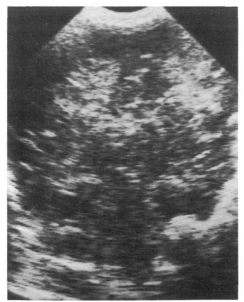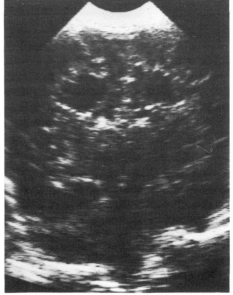

Fig. 6.5. Resolution of periventricular echodensity *(left)*, to extensive cystic degeneration *(right)* over the course of three weeks.

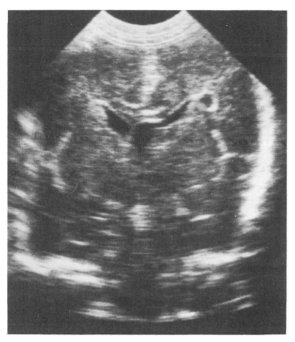

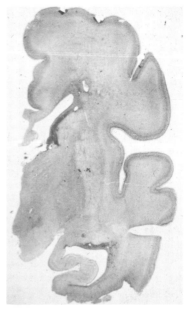

Fig. 6.6. Single right-sided periventricular cyst detected on coronal scan.

Fig. 6.7. Section through right hemisphere in infant illustrated in Figure 6.6, showing the discrete cyst at the lateral-most margin of right lateral ventricle.

both coronal and parasagittal planes (Fig. 6.3). On microscopic examination, these echogenic areas correspond to fresh necrosis with pyknosis and sponginess. This is associated with either a marked vascular congestion and/or secondary bleeding within the focus of necrosis.

The reason for the periventricular echodensity in the early stages of PVL is not completely clear. Grant *et al.* (1983) described a periventricular echogenic halo particularly in the area of the splenium posteriorly in almost 180 consecutively scanned infants, and there is no doubt that this is a normal appearance. In only two infants, however, was this echodense appearance seen in both coronal and parasagittal planes, and in both cases ischaemic or haemorrhagic infarction was suspected. We would agree that the diagnosis of PVL at this stage of its evolution may be extremely difficult, but important features include the extent of the echodense areas. Those extending more anteriorly are likely to be more significant. In addition, recognition in coronal and parasagittal planes is essential; the more intense it is, the more likely it is that this is due to haemorrhagic infarction or venous congestion. We have seen one infant with periventricular echoes who at post-mortem had marked venous infarction in this region (Fig. 6.4). This was due to superior sagittal sinus thrombosis, which was not detected by ultrasound.

Sequential ultrasound scanning has defined the sequence of changes in these lesions. Areas of increased echodensity resolve into echo-free areas that

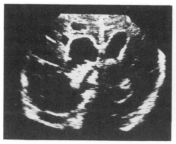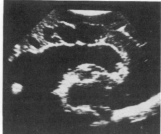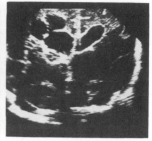

Fig. 6.8. Multiple cysts in periventricular region on coronal and parasagittal scans. Although there may be some communication with ventricular system, ependyma is largely intact. Intraventricular haemorrhage is also present.

progressively increase in size and become well circumscribed (Fig. 6.5). The final stage is a cyst which does not appear to communicate with the ventricular system in the majority of cases (Figs. 6.6 to 6.8). The cystic degeneration is characterised on microscopy by an astrocytic reaction, proliferation of microglia and accumulation of lipid-laden macrophages in the necrotic tissue (Fig. 6.2). In severe cases, reduction of the volume of the hemispheric white matter may be noted; this appears on ultrasound as an enlargement of the interhemispheric fissure. We have noted that in a number of infants, these periventricular cysts are no longer seen on ultrasound scan by six months of age. The reason for this is not clear.

A number of conditions associated with cavitation show the same predilection for the periventricular tissue. The following points may be of help in identifying the nature of the cystic lesions. Periventricular leukomalacia are recognisable by their often bilateral distribution around (but separate from) the lateral margins of the ventricles. Cysts resulting from neonatal meningitis produce larger cavities in a more random distribution, which are often associated with cortical lesions (Fig. 9.7). The cortex and other parts of the brain are commonly spared in PVL occurring in premature infants. Cavitation due to parenchymal extension of germinal layer haemorrhage usually opens into the ventricular system (Fig. 6.9). The latter entity must be distinguished from cystic PVL lesions as they both may occur in premature infants, but their respective aetiologies are ascribed to different pathophysiological mechanisms (Pape and Wigglesworth 1979).

Hypoxic-ischaemic lesions in the term infant

As described in the introduction, various patterns of cerebral damage occur in the mature neonate. Several animal studies have been reported which elucidate pathophysiological and anatomical mechanisms leading to brain injury (Myers 1975). Term monkey fetuses subjected to episodes of partial asphyxia showed lesions mainly affecting the cerebral hemispheres. The damage, when severe, consisted of a total cortical necrosis. With less severe injury, the lesion might be restricted to the middle third of the paracentral region, or to the basal ganglia. After a period of total asphyxia, term monkey fetuses exhibited damage mainly in the region of the brainstem. In the term human neonate, however, a mixed pattern

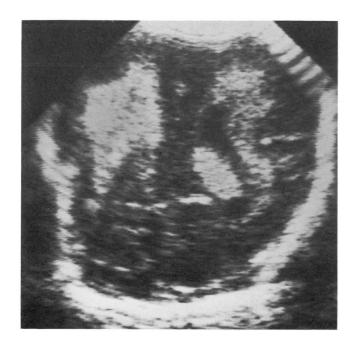

Fig. 6.9. Co-existence of extensive haemorrhage together with periventricular leukomalacia. **(a)** Coronal scan, showing left-sided parenchymal haemorrhage, with less echodensity in periventricular region of the right ventricle.

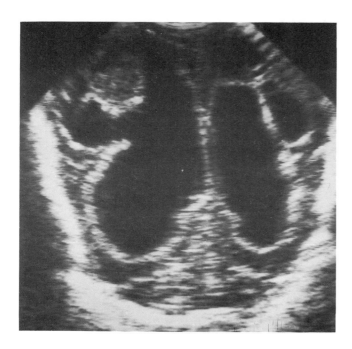

Fig. 6.9b. Two weeks later, a porencephalic cyst had developed in left hemisphere, freely communicating with the left ventricle. In right hemisphere, a number of periventricular cysts have developed.

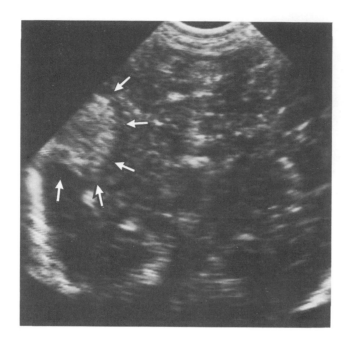

Fig. 6.10. Middle cerebral artery infarction in term infant. Coronal view **(a)** showing a well-circumscribed echodense area *(arrowed)* obscuring insula in region supplied by left middle cerebral artery.

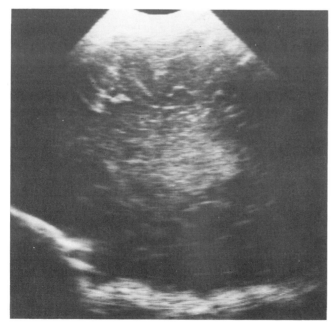

Fig. 6.10b. Extreme parasagittal scan shows this echodense area in the region of the insula.

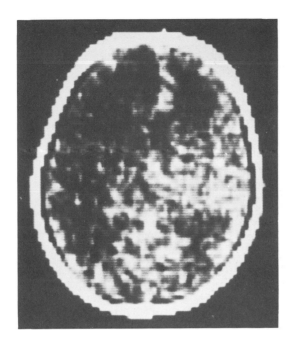

Fig. 6.11. Computerised X-ray tomogram on same infant as shown in Figure 6.10. There is increased attenuation corresponding with middle cerebral artery infarction.

of lesions is quite often noted, usually with predominance of one or other type (Towbin 1969, Friede 1975).

Boundary zone infarction, PVL and subcortial leukomalacia
Infarction may be noted involving the cortex and the white matter at the watershed regions between the territories of the anterior, middle and posterior cerebral arteries, and less commonly in the mature infant at the boundary zones in the periventricular white matter between the central and the cortical arterial supplies. Post-mortem cerebral angiography (Takashima *et al.* 1978) has shown the development of the microvascular architecture of the cerebral cortex and the white matter. In the more mature brain, a relatively avascular triangle forms in the white matter at the depth of the sulcus and could explain the different site of ischaemic lesion among term infants.

Hill *et al.* (1983) have recently described four cases of focal echogenic areas corresponding to the areas of low attenuation seen on computerised x-ray tomography. These are thought to represent areas of ischaemic injury (Flodmark *et al.* 1980, Volpe 1981), and the territory of the middle cerebral artery is frequently involved (Barmada *et al.* 1979, O'Brien *et al.* 1979, Hill *et al.* 1983). It is sometimes possible to observe changes in arterial pulsations on real-time scanning with reduced pulsating echoes originating from affected arteries (Hill *et al.* 1983). It is still unclear why ischaemic damage should appear on ultrasound as echodense areas. Hill *et al.* (1983) apparently exclude oedema as a cause, and speculate that a decrease in tissue fluid would produce increased echodensity. An alternative

85

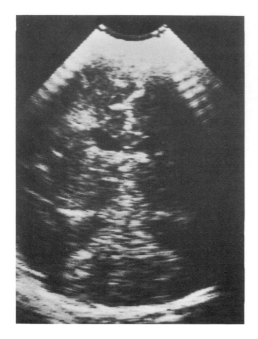

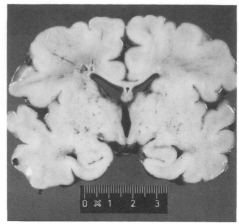

Fig. 6.12. *Left:* coronal ultrasound scan from a term infant showing periventricular echodensity. *Above:* area of PVL seen at post-mortem examination.

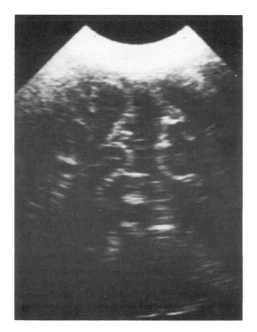

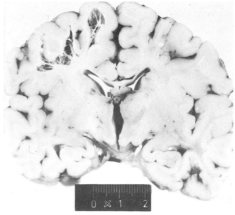

Fig. 6.13. *Left:* subcortical cystic degeneration with marked separation of inter-hemispheric fissure suggesting cerebral atrophy. *Above:* post-mortem specimen showing extensive subcortical cysts.

explanation is that ischaemic lesions may be associated with vascular congestion and tissue sponginess. The latter features sufficiently alter tissue characteristics thus producing multiple small interfaces resulting in increased echo-reflectance. Very few ultrasound reports have been published up to now describing this type of injury. In one case, scanning revealed areas of increased echodensity involving the white matter and cerebral cortex in the region of the arterial supply of one of the major cerebral arteries (Figs. 6.10 and 6.11). Although PVL occurs most often among preterm infants, it has also been reported in term infants (Armstrong and Norman 1974, Fawer *et al.* 1983). The ultrasound appearance is similar, with areas of increased echodensity in the periventricular white matter (Fig. 6.12).

Periventricular and subcortical leukomalacia are both attributed to cerebral underperfusion. They are related to the state of maturity of the vascular supply and to the sites of vascular watershed (Norman 1949, Banker and Larroche 1962, De Reuck 1971). Periventricular leukomalacia occurs at the watershed between ventriculopetal and ventriculofugal arteries. Subcortical leukomalacia is most prominent at the watersheds between the major cerebral arteries, and at watershed zones at the depth of the sulci in term infants (Figs. 6.13 and 6.15). The ultrasound appearances are identical to those in premature infants with increased echodensity in the early stage, and cyst formation later. Their respective topography depends on the type of ischaemic damage.

Twins, especially the monozygotic variety, are well known to have an increased risk of cerebral lesions (Aicardi *et al.* 1972, Schinzel *et al.* 1979, Yoshioka *et al.* 1979). These have been assumed to be due to disturbances in their shared circulation together with other complications including disseminated intravascular coagulation and thrombo-embolism (Moore *et al.* 1969). These lesions have also been reported to occur *in utero* in the twin of a macerated fetus. In one surviving twin, ultrasound examination revealed multiple cystic cavities with large septa occurring in the white matter of both hemispheres (Fig. 6.15).

Lesions of the thalami
These lesions occur in infants following acute episodes of total asphyxia. Similar damage has been produced in animal studies (Windle *et al.* 1962, Myers 1975) following sudden clamping of the umbilical cord. The thalami and brainstem nuclei bear the brunt of this insult because of their high metabolic requirements (Myers 1975).

The ultrasound appearances of this particular type of ischaemic damage have been poorly documented. In one case scanned shortly after birth, focal areas of highly increased echodensity, located in the basal ganglia and associated with subependymal pseudocysts and dilated ventricles, were seen (Fig. 6.16). At necropsy, extensive microcalcification in the pallidum and thalami was noted. Intra-uterine infection was excluded. This infant probably suffered a severe episode of asphyxia *in utero* associated with the development of acute polyhydramnios, and at birth failed to establish spontaneous respiration. Clearly, further studies with neuropathological correlation are needed to identify specific ischaemic lesions occurring in term infants. Brainstem nuclei and the other sites involved in this type

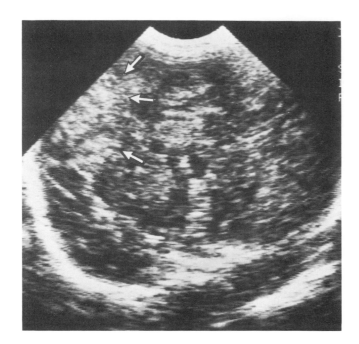

Fig. 6.14. Subcortical leukomalacia in a term infant. **(a)** Coronal *(above)* scan showing echodensities in subcortical area *(arrowed)*.

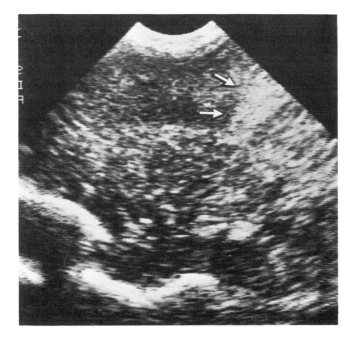

Fig. 6.14b. Parasagittal scan showing echodensities in subcortical area *(arrowed)*.

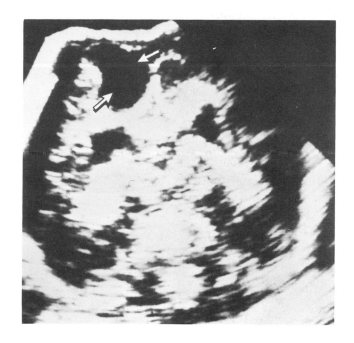

Fig. 6.15a. Coronal scan showing multiple subcortical cystic cavities *(arrows)* in a surviving twin.

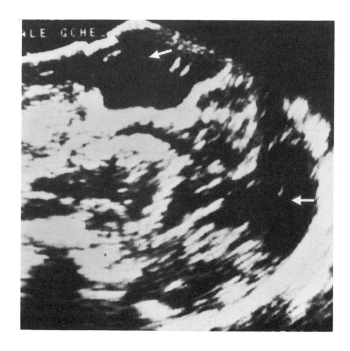

Fig. 6.15b. Parasagittal scan showing multiple subcortical cystic cavities *(arrows)* in a surviving twin.

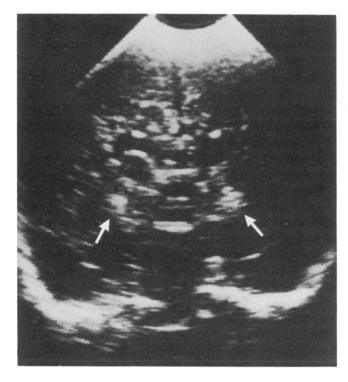

Fig. 6.16. Basal ganglia calcification. Coronal scan from a full-term infant showing discrete areas of thalamic echo-genicity *(arrows)* together with a subependymal pseudocyst. Histology revealed the thalamic lesions to be due to microcalcification.

of insult are incompletely visualised by ultrasound, and damage to these areas may only be detected with difficulty.

Status marmaratus of the basal ganglia is a well-known neuropathological entity (Norman 1949, Malamud 1950). Its true frequency is not known, but its relationship to perinatal asphyxia in term infants is well established. Myers (1969) produced similar lesions in his animal models, and the characteristic lesions consisted of abnormal patterns of myelination with extensive glial reaction which took several months to develop fully. By the time this lesion is fully evolved, the size of the anterior fontanelle in the human infant may make intracranial examination difficult, and for this reason these lesions may not be fully appreciated.

The perinatal brain is vulnerable to many insults which may or may not cause structural brain damage. In turn, the structural damage may subsequently be associated with functional disability. Such 'pure' pathophysiological reactions, as described in this section, may be recognisable on ultrasound examination. The brain, however, may eventually show signs of gross cerebral atrophy, making the distinction of original aetiology impossible. The ultrasound appearances of cerebral atrophy are discussed in Chapter 10. Other lesions associated with ischaemia and hypoxia in the developing brain are discussed elsewhere, including porencephaly, hydranencephaly (Chapter 7) and cerebral oedema (Chapter 10).

REFERENCES

Aicardi, J., Goutières, F., de Verbois, A. H. (1972) 'Multicystic encephalomalacia of infants and its relation to abnormal gestation and hydranencephaly.' *Journal of the Neurological Sciences,* **15,** 357.

Armstrong, D., Norman, M. G. (1974) 'Periventricular leukomalacia in neonates: complications and sequelae.' *Archives of Disease in Childhood,* **49,** 367-375.

Banker, B. Q., Larroche, J. C. (1962) 'Periventricular leukomalacia of infancy: a form of neonatal anoxic encephalopathy.' *Archives of Neurology,* **7,** 386-410.

Barmada, M. A., Moossy, J., Shuman, R. M. (1979) 'Cerebral infarcts with arterial occlusion in neonates.' *Annals of Neurology,* **6,** 495-502.

Brown, J. K., Purvis, R. J., Fortar, J. O., Cockburn, F (1974) 'Neurological aspects of perinatal asphyxia.' *Developmental Medicine and Child Neurology,* **16,** 567-580.

Couture, A., Cadier, L. (1983) *Echographie Cérébrale par Voie Transfontanellaire.* Paris: Vigot.

De Reuck, J. (1971) 'The human periventricular arterial blood supply and the anatomy of cerebral infarctions.' *European Neurology,* **5,** 321-334.

—— Chattha, A. S., Richardson, E. P. (1972) 'Pathogenesis and evolution of periventricular leukomalacia in infancy.' *Archives of Neurology,* **27,** 229-236.

Di Chiro, G., Arimitsu, R., Pellock, J. M., Landes, R. D. (1978) 'Periventricular leukomalacia related to neonatal anoxia: recognition by computed tomography.' *Journal of Computer Assisted Tomography,* **2,** 352-355.

Estrada, M., El Gammal, T., Dyken, P. R. (1980) 'Periventricular low attenuations. A normal finding in computerized tomographic scans of neonates?' *Archives of Neurology,* **37,** 754-756.

Fawer, C.-L., Calame, A., Perentes, E., Anderegg, A. (1985) 'Periventricular leukomalacia: a correlation study between real-time ultrasound and autopsy findings.' *(Submitted for publication.)*

Flodmark, O., Fitz, R., Harwood-Nash, D. C. (1980) 'CT diagnosis and short-term prognosis of intracranial hemorrhage and hypoxic-ischemic brain damage in neonates.' *Journal of Computer Assisted Tomography,* **4,** 775-785.

Friede, R. L. (1975) *Developmental Neuropathology.* Vienna: Springer. p. 44.

Grant, E. G., Schellinger, D., Richardson, J. D., Coffey, M. L., Smirniotopoulous, J. G. (1983) 'Echogenic periventricular halo: normal sonographic finding or neonatal cerebral hemorrhage.' *American Journal of Neuroradiology,* **4,** 43-46.

Hambleton, G., Wigglesworth, J. S. (1976) 'Origin of intraventricular haemorrhage in the preterm infant.' *Archives of Disease in Childhood,* **51,** 651-659.

Hill, A., Melson, G. L., Clark, H. B., Volpe, J. J. (1982) 'Hemorrhagic periventricular leukomalacia: diagnosis by real-time ultrasound and correlation with autopsy findings.' *Pediatrics,* **69,** 282-284.

—— Martin, D. J., Daneman, A., Fitz, C. R. (1983) 'Focal ischemic cerebral injury in the newborn: diagnosis by ultrasound and correlation with computed tomographic scan.' *Pediatrics,* **71,** 790-793.

Hirabayashi, S., Kitahara, T., Hishiba, T. (1980) 'Computer tomography in perinatal hypoxic and hypoglycemie encephalopathy with emphasis on follow-up studies.' *Journal of Computer Assisted Tomography,* **4,** 451-456.

Leech, R. W., Alvord, E. C. (1974) 'Morphologic variations in periventricular leukomalacia.' *American Journal of Pathology,* **74,** 591-602.

Levene, M. I., Wigglesworth, J. S., Dubowitz, V. (1983) 'Haemorrhagic periventricular leukomalacia in the neonate: a real-time ultrasound study.' *Pediatrics,* **71,** 794-797.

Malamud, N. (1950) 'Status marmoratus. A form of cerebral palsy following either birth injury or inflammation of the central nervous system.' *Journal of Pediatrics,* **37,** 610-619.

Moore, C. M., McAdams, A. J., Sutherland, J. (1969) 'Intrauterine disseminated intravascular coagulation: a syndrome of multiple pregnancy with dead twin fetus.' *Journal of Pediatrics,* **74,** 523-528.

Myers, R. E. (1969) 'Atrophic cortical sclerosis associated with status marmoratus in a perinatally damaged monkey.' *Neurology,* **19,** 1177-1188.

—— (1975) 'Fetal asphyxia due to umbilical cord compression: metabolic and brain pathologic consequences.' *Biology of the Neonate,* **26,** 21-43.

Norman, R. M. (1949) 'Etat marbré of the thalamus following birth injury.' *Brain,* **72,** 83-88.

O'Brien, M. J., Ash, M. J., Gilday, D. L. (1979) 'Radionuclide brain scanning in perinatal hypoxia-ischemia.' *Developmental Medicine and Child Neurology,* **21,** 161-173.

Pape, K. E., Wigglesworth, J. S. (1979) *Haemorrhage, Ischaemia and the Perinatal Brain. Clinics in Developmental Medicine No. 69/70.* London: SIMP with Heinemann; Philadelphia: Lippincott.

Parrot, J. (1873) 'Etude sur le ramollissement de l'encéphale chez le nouveau-né.' *Archives de*

91

Physiologie Normale et Pathologique, **5,** 59-73, 176-95, 283-303.

Schinzel, A. G., Smith, D. W., Miller, J. R. (1979) 'Monozygotic twinning and structural defects.' *Journal of Pediatrics,* **95,** 921-930.

Shuman, R. M., Selednik, L. J. (1980) 'Periventricular leukomalacia. A one-year autopsy study.' *Archives of Neurology,* **37,** 231-235.

Smith, J. F., Reynolds, E. O. R., Taghizadeh, A. (1974) 'Brain maturation and damage in infants dying from chronic pulmonary insufficiency in the postnatal period.' *Archives of Disease in Childhood,* **49,** 359-366.

Takashima, S., Armstrong, D. L., Becker, L. E. (1978) 'Subcortical leukomalacia.' *Archives of Neurology,* **35,** 470-472.

Towbin, A. (1969) 'Cerebral hypoxic damage in fetus and newborn.' *Archives of Neurology,* **20,** 35-43.

Virchow, R. (1867) 'Zur pathologischen Anatomie des Gehirns. 1. Congenitale Encephalitis und Myelitis.' *Virchows Archives für Pathologische Anatomie,* **38,** 129-142.

Volpe, J. J. (1976) 'Perinatal hypoxic-ischemic brain injury.' *Pediatric Clinics of North America,* **23,** 383-397.

—— (1981) 'Neurology of the newborn.' *Major Problems in Clinical Pediatrics,* **22,** 141-179.

Wigglesworth, J. S., Pape, K. E. (1978) 'An integrated model for haemorrhagic and ischemic lesions in the newborn brain.' *Early Human Development,* **2,** 179-199.

Windle, W. F., Jacobson, H. N., Robert de Raminez de Arellano, M. I., Combs, C. M. (1962) 'Structure and functional sequelae of asphyxia neonatorum in monkeys (Macaca mulatta).' *Research Publications of the Association for Research into Nervous and Mental Disorders,* **39,** 169-182.

Yoshioka, H., Kadamoto, Y., Mino, H., Morikawa, Y., Kasubichi, Y., Kusunoki, T. (1979) 'Multicystic encephalomalacia in a liveborn twin with a stillborn macerated twin.' *Journal of Pediatrics,* **95,** 798-800.

Ziegler, A. L., Calame, A., Marchand, D., Passera, M., Reymond-Goni, I., Prod'hom, L. S. (1976) 'Cerebral distress in full-term newborns and its prognostic value: a follow-up study of 90 infants.' *Helvetica Paediatrica Acta,* **31,** 299-317.

7
INTRACRANIAL CYSTS

Intracranial cysts are fluid-filled sacs within the cranium that displace adjacent parenchyma to produce a mass effect. The fluid may be normal cerebrospinal fluid (CSF), inflammatory transudate, or may contain a high concentration of protein. Cysts with a fluid that has a high protein content may be the result of parenchymal infection (Grant *et al.* 1982) with or without haemorrhage, infection (Stannard and Jimenez 1983) or tumours with a cystic component (Sauerbrei and Cooperberg 1983, Smith *et al.* 1983).

Hydranencephaly
This is the complete absence of the hemispheric parenchyma due to early intra-uterine occlusion of both internal carotid arteries. This occlusion occurs in the supraclinoid or proximal intracranial portion of the internal carotid arteries (Babcock and Han 1981). The residual mantle is a thin membrane, and is little more than the meninges with a few glial elements. Only that portion of the brain supplied by the posterior cerebral circulation remains. This includes the brainstem, a portion of the occipital lobes, the hypothalamus and the basal ganglia. There is usually preservation of the falx (Figs. 7.1 to 7.3).

Severe hydrocephalus or ventricular enlargement can result in an appearance

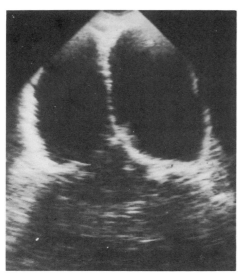 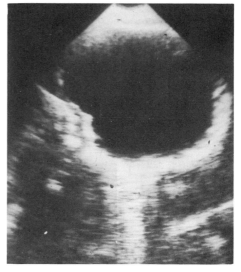

Fig. 7.1. Hydranencephaly in an infant born at term following congenital cytomegalovirus infection. *Left:* coronal scan showing total absence of cerebral tissue with only a vestigial midline echo. *Right:* parasagittal scan from same infant showing no echoes from within skull. (Reproduced by courtesy of Dr. Linda de Vries.)

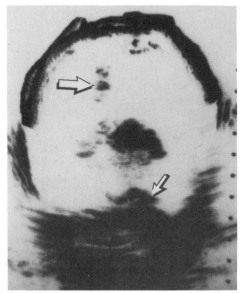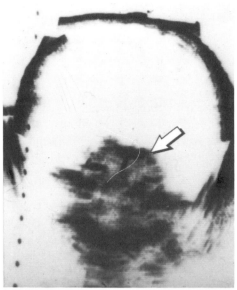

Fig. 7.2. Hydranencephaly. *Above left:* coronal B-scan demonstrates irregular tissue in the posterior fossa *(arrow)*. Paramidline echoes suggest the present of a septum *(small arrow)*. *Above right:* coronal B-scan angled slightly more posteriorly and showing fused midline thalami *(arrow)*. Brainstem is just inferior to basal ganglia. These features indicate absence of parenchyma supplied by internal carotid arteries.

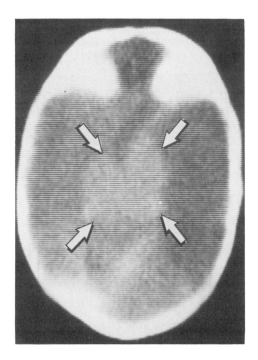

Fig. 7.3. *(left):* hydranencephaly. An axial CT scan from same infant illustrated in Figure 7.2. This shows fused basal ganglia *(arrows)*. No residual brain parenchyma is present, and vault is filled with CSF.

94

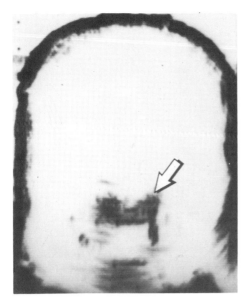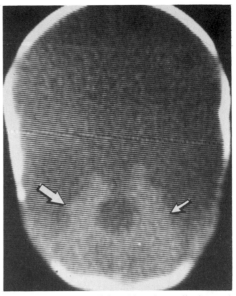

Fig. 7.4. Severe hydrocephalus. *Above left:* axial B-scan also showing small fused basal ganglia *(arrow)*, but there is no occipital tissue present in the posterior fossa. *Above right:* CT scan showing tissue remaining only around brainstem *(arrows)*; again no occipital mantle is present.

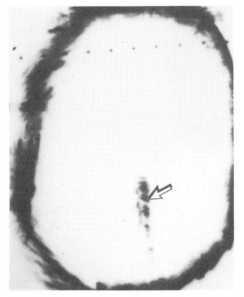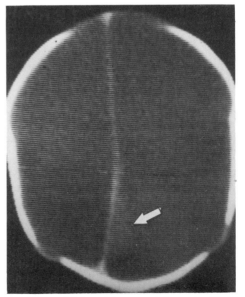

Fig. 7.5. Severe hydrocephalus. *Above left:* this B-scan shows a faint septal remnant *(arrow)* with no peripheral parenchyma. *Above right:* axial CT better demonstrates the remaining midline falx with minimal dysmorphic tissue adjacent to it *(arrow)*.

95

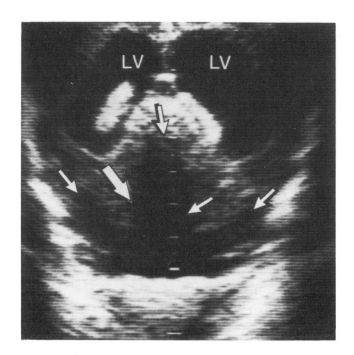

Fig. 7.6. Dandy-Walker cyst. **(a)** Coronal sonogram demonstrates bilateral lateral ventricular (LV) enlargement. A large bell-shaped cyst *(arrows)* fills midline in posterior fossa.

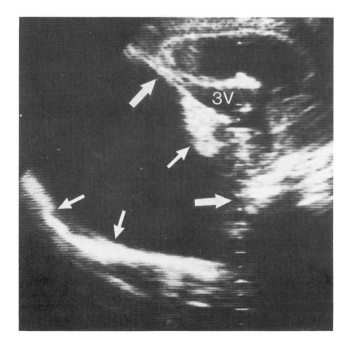

Fig. 7.6b. Sagittal sonogram illustrates massive dilatation of fourth ventricle *(arrows)* with no cerebellar vermis remaining. Third ventricle (3V) is moderately prominent.

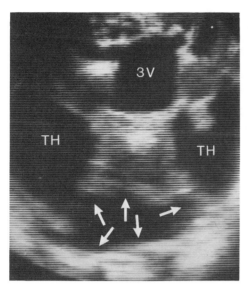

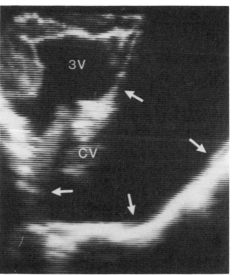

Fig. 7.7. Dandy-Walker variant. Coronal sonogram shows elevation of large third ventricle (3V) due to absence of corpus callosum. Temporal horns (TH) are very large and are laterally placed. Midline cyst fills posterior fossa *(arrows)*.

Fig. 7.8. Dandy-Walker variant. Sagittal sonogram shows enlarged and deformed third ventricle (3V). Large cyst in posterior fossa *(arrows)* is posterior and inferior to small echogenic cerebellar vermis (CV).

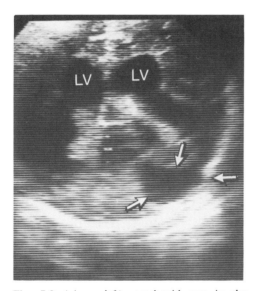

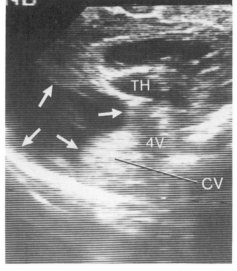

Fig. 7.9 *(above left)*: arachnoid cyst in the posterior fossa. The coronal sonogram illustrates lateral ventricular enlargement (LV). A cyst is seen within the posterior fossa, to left of midline *(arrows)*.

Fig. 7.10 *(above right)*: arachnoid cyst in posterior fossa. Parasagittal sonogram demonstrates an elevated temporal horn (TH) of lateral ventricle. Vermis of cerebellum (CV) is normal and is bounded posteriorly by separate arachnoid cyst *(arrows)*. There is preservation of fourth ventricle (4V).

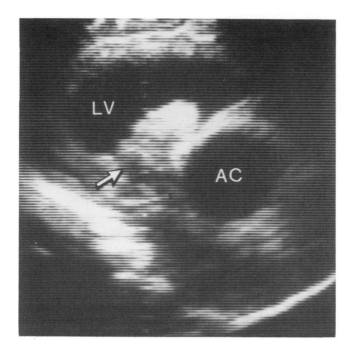

Fig. 7.11. Arachnoid cyst arising from third ventricle. A sagittal sonogram demonstrates a large lateral ventricle (LV). Just posterior to a relatively small and obstructed third ventricle *(arrow)* is a large arachnoid cyst (AC). In this patient, there was a history of meningitis and the aetiology of the pial entrapment was thought to be inflammatory.

similar to the hydranencephalic brain (Figs. 7.4 and 7.5). In this case, however, there is little or no preservation of the occipital lobes. Angiography can be performed to demonstrate complete absence of internal carotid arteries (hydranencephaly) or stretching and attenuation of these arteries (severe ventricular enlargement or hydrocephalus). Distinction between these two entities has little clinical importance.

Dandy-Walker cysts

Cystic lesions in the posterior fossa are generally grouped under the heading of Dandy-Walker cysts (Raybaud 1982, Grant *et al.* 1983). Three separate subdivisions occur, and all can be associated with the following supratentorial malformations: a single ventricle (holoprosencephaly), absence of the corpus callosum, and cysts in the thalamic-hypothalamic regions.

A true Dandy-Walker malformation results from atresia of the foramen of Magendie and usually the foramina of Luschka as well. In addition, there is partial agenesis of the cerebellar vermis. This results in massive dilatation of the fourth ventricle and less prominent enlargement of the third and lateral ventricles (Fig. 7.6).

The Dandy-Walker variant has an identical appearance and dysplasia of the cerebellar vermis is also present. There is, however, communication into the perimedullary spaces through a patent foramen of Magendie. The fourth ventricle is separate and is less dilated (Figs. 7.7 and 7.8).

Arachnoid pouches, cysts of the retrocerebellar space, cisterna magna cysts or

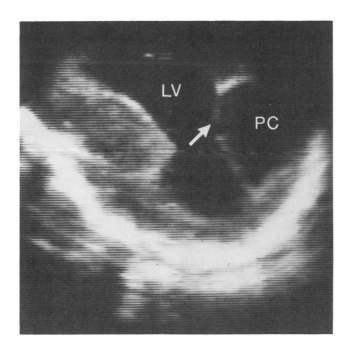

Fig. 7.12. Porencephalic cyst. Parasagittal sonogram showing enlarged lateral ventricle (LV). Communicating through a cleft *(arrow)* is a large cyst (PC). Several weeks prior to this scan, patient had an intraparenchymal haemorrhage in region of the cyst.

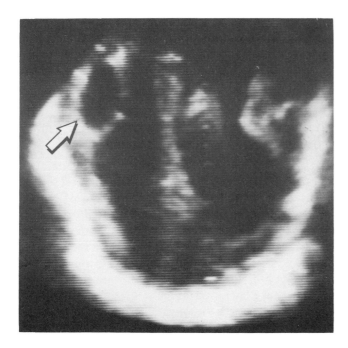

Fig. 7.13. Porencephalic cyst. A semi-axial sonogram showing extensive cerebral parenchymal loss from a previous haemorrhage. A relatively small porencephalic cyst *(arrow)* is seen laterally, communicating with lateral ventricle.

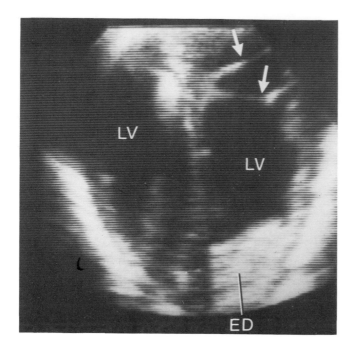

Fig. 7.14. Inflammatory porencephalic cysts. A coronal sonogram illustrates multiple membranes or synechia *(arrows)* secondary to extensive cerebritis and marked ventricular enlargement (LV). Echogenic debris (ED) lies dependently in left occipital horn.

Blake's pouch deformity comprise the third type of lesion that presents with a posterior fossa cyst. Here there is a normal fourth ventricle with no abnormality of the vermis (Figs. 7.9 and 7.10). Similar associated supratentorial abnormalities can be found. As in the Dandy-Walker variant, there is often a communication with the subarachnoid spaces. Elevation of the torcular Herophili can be found in all three variations, indicating the congenital origin of the malformations.

Arachnoid cysts

Cysts of the arachnoid usually occur when there is a congenital invagination or inflammatory entrapment of this pial layer. They occur most commonly around the sella turcica, basilar cisterns and as a posterior extension from the roof of the third ventricle (Fig. 7.11). These cysts contain normal cerebrospinal fluid and produce symptoms by displacement of adjacent normal brain (Haller and Shkolnik 1981). In the presence of severe hydrocephalus, there is occasionally herniation of the arachnoid through the inferior-medial wall of the trigone (Naidich *et al.* 1982). This lateral ventricular pulsion diverticulum may herniate below the tentorium and compress the structures in the posterior fossa, including the brainstem and cerebellum. Rarely, a suboccipital dermal sinus may lead into an intracranial cyst in the posterior fossa.

Porencephalic cysts

These contain CSF and usually communicate with the ventricles or the subarachnoid spaces. While such cysts may be developmental due to incomplete closure of the telencephalon, they are more commonly the result of acquired focal parenchymal loss. Trauma, infection, infarction and haemorrhage are the usual causes of such localized brain destruction (Figs. 7.12 and 7.13).

Clinical and experimental evolution of both abscess formation and intra-parenchymal haemorrhage is well documented (Enzmann *et al.* 1982). Initially there is a homogeneously echogenic lesion. This evolves into a structure with a hypoechoic centre and a hyperechoic periphery which reflects resolution and glial repair. Removal of residual débris completes the encephaloclastic porencephalic cyst formation (Fig. 7.14). There is often associated ventricular enlargement. With shunting, the porencephalic cyst may either reduce in size or remain the same.

Other cystic lesions

Primary brain tumours (Chapter 10) are rare in the newborn or infant (Sauerbrei and Cooperberg 1983, Smith *et al.* 1983). A cystic component may be present in the tumour. Vascular malformations, such as a vein of Galen aneurysm (Chapter 8), also appear as cysts and may not pulsate on real-time examination. Their location, posterior to the third ventricle, may aid in the diagnosis (Sivakoff and Nouri 1982, Rodemyer and Smith 1982).

REFERENCES

Babcock, D. S., Han, B. K. (1981) *Cranial Ultrasonography of Infants.* Baltimore: Williams & Wilkins. pp. 152-172.

Enzmann, D. R., Britt, R. H., Lyons, B., Carroll, B., Wilson, D. A., Buxton, J. (1982) 'High-resolution ultrasound evaluation of experimental brain abscess evolution: comparison with computed tomography and neuropathology.' *Radiology,* **142,** 95-102.

Grant, E. G., Kerner, M., Schellinger, D., Borts, F. T., McCullough, D. C., Smith, Y., Sivasubramanian, K. N., Davitt, M. K. (1982) 'Evolution of porencephalic cysts from intra-parenchymal hemorrhage in neonates: sonographic evidence.' *American Journal of Roentgenology,* **138,** 467-470 (see also: *American Journal of Neuroradiology,* **3,** 47-50).

Grant, E. G., Schellinger, D., Richardson, J. D. (1983) 'Real-time ultrasonography of the posterior fossa.' *Journal of Ultrasound in Medicine,* **2,** 73-87.

Haller, J. O., Shkolnik, A. (1981) *Ultrasound in Pediatrics. Clinics in Diagnostic Ultrasound No. 8.* Edinburgh: Churchill Livingstone. pp. 13-27.

Naidich, T. P., McLone, D. G., Hahn, Y. S., Hanaway, J. (1982) 'Atrial diverticula in severe hydrocephalus.' *American Journal of Neuroradiology,* **3,** 257-266.

Raybaud, C. (1982) 'Cystic malformations of the posterior fossa.' *Journal of Neuroradiology,* **9,** 103-133.

Rodemyer, C. R., Smith, W. L. (1982) 'Diagnosis of a vein of Galen aneurysm by ultrasound.' *Journal of Clinical Ultrasound,* **10,** 297-298.

Sauerbrei, E. E., Cooperberg, P. L. (1983) 'Cystic tumors of the fetal and neonatal cerebrum: ultrasound and computed tomographic evaluation.' *Radiology,* **147,** 689-692.

Sivakoff, M., Nouri, S. (1982) 'Diagnosis of vein of Galen arteriovenous malformation by two-dimensional ultrasound and pulsed Doppler method.' *Pediatrics,* **69,** 84-86.

Smith, W. L., Menezes, A., Franken, E. A. (1983) 'Cranial ultrasound in the diagnosis of malignant brain tumors.' *Journal of Clinical Ultrasound,* **11,** 97-100.

Stannard, M. W., Jimenez, J. F. (1983) 'Sonographic recognition of multiple cystic encephalomalacia.' *American Journal of Roentgenology,* **141,** 1321-1324 (see also: *American Journal of Neuroradiology,* **4,** 1111-1114).

8
NON-CYSTIC CONGENITAL ABNORMALITIES

In this chapter we will consider abnormalities of cerebral development, other than those of a cystic nature. The development of the brain and spinal cord is an extremely complicated process which continues into the second decade before final maturity is achieved. Abnormalities in the development of the central nervous system (CNS) are common, and up to 75 per cent of fetal deaths and 40 per cent of deaths in infancy are due to CNS malformations (Adams and Sidman 1968). Furthermore, one third of all congenital abnormalities identified in the perinatal period arise from the central nervous system (Menkes 1974). These abnormalities are often evident at birth, but some cerebral malformations may not be immediately obvious. The infant with dysmorphic features or abnormal neuro-logical behaviour may suggest cerebral malformations, and various imaging techniques are essential for further clarification. Due to the wide spectrum of congenital CNS abnormalities, only the more common ones amenable to ultrasound diagnosis will be discussed here.

Holoprosencephaly
This is a rare condition, which is due to failure of the primary cerebral vesicle to split and develop bilaterally. The brain has a single midline ventricular cavity, fused thalami and rudimentary cortical mantle. Other associated major cerebral

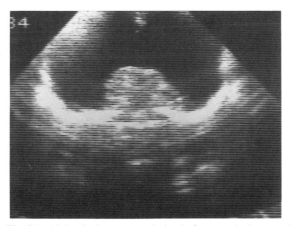
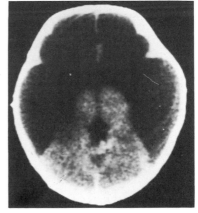

Fig. 8.1. Alobar holoprosencephaly. *Left:* coronal ultrasound scan through middle cranial fossa showing a central portion of cerebral tissue surrounded by echo-free fluid. *Right:* computerised axial tomogram of same infant confirming absence of cerebral tissue in the frontal and temporoparietal regions of the brain.

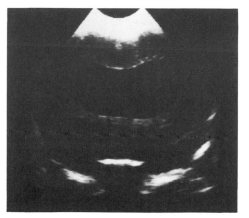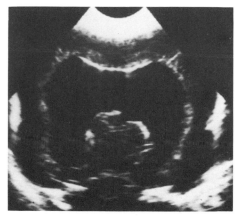

Fig. 8.2. Lobar holoprosencephaly in infant with arrhinencephaly. *Left:* mid-coronal scan showing a single midline ventricle with no evidence of septum pellucidum. *Right:* posterior coronal scan showing fusion of occipital horns in midline.

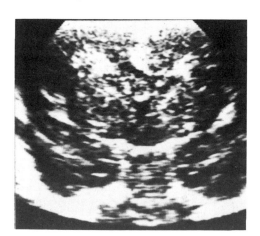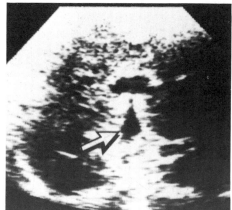

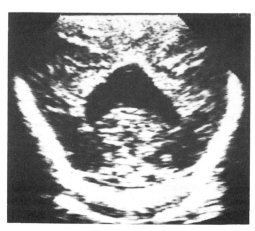

Fig. 8.3. Semi-lobar holoprosencephaly. Serial coronal scans from anterior *(above left)* to posterior *(left)*, showing fusion of ventricles in midline with an abnormally placed third ventricle *(arrowed)*.

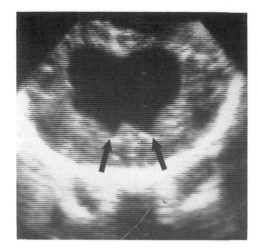

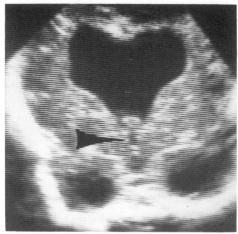

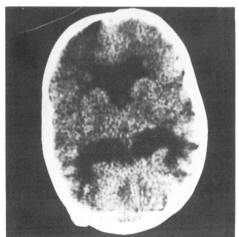

Fig. 8.4 *(above left):* septo-optic dysplasia. Large lateral ventricles on coronal scan, with no evidence of septum pellucidum. There is inferior pointing in the floor of anterior poles of the lateral ventricles *(arrows).*

Fig. 8.5. *(above right):* septo-optic dysplasia. Dilated lateral ventricles with small dysmorphic third ventricle. Midline septum pellucidum could not be visualised.

Fig. 8.6 *(left):* septo-optic dysplasia. Axial CT scan of the same infant illustrated in Figure 8.5 showing this condition.

malformations such as ethmocephaly and cebocephaly are always present. This condition may be associated with trisomy 13 to 15, and affected infants have a characteristic appearance often with midline facial clefts. This malformation is incompatible with prolonged survival.

Holoprosencephaly can be divided into degrees of severity and referred to as alobar and lobar. In the less severe lobar variety there is only incomplete cleavage. The ultrasound of the alobar variety is characteristic and shows a large central echo-free ventricle. The cortical mantle is often extremely thinned, and appears to be present only as a rim at the base of the anterior and middle fossae (Fig. 8.1). The infratentorial structures are usually present, and should be recognised sonographically. The lobar form occurs more commonly and shows more complete separation into lateral ventricles. Fusion of the anterior or occipital horns is present, and there is an incomplete septum pellucidum (Fig. 8.2). In even less severe forms there may

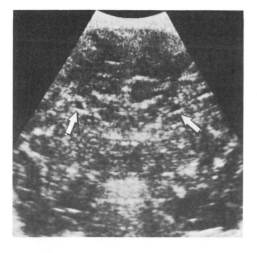
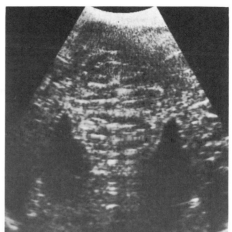
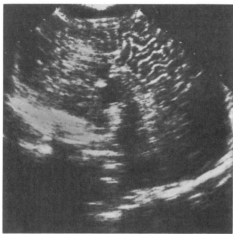

Fig. 8.7. Agenesis of the corpus callosum *(above left and right)*. Lateral ventricles *(arrowed)* are widely separated on coronal scans. *Left:* on parasagittal section, the corpus callosum cannot be visualised. In addition there are echogenic structures radiating posteriorly.

only be partial division of the hemispheres (Fig. 8.3), and the olfactory bulbs and nerves are absent—this form is called arrhinencephaly. It is unlikely that ultrasound alone will diagnose this condition.

Septo-optic dysplasia

This is a midline defect of the brain associated with optic nerve hypoplasia. Characteristically this condition includes absence of the septum pellucidum, malformation of the forebrain, and hypothalamic-pituitary dysfunction. The appearances are shown in Figures 8.4 to 8.6. Other associated abnormalities include cleft lip and palate, together with absence of olfactory bulbs and tracts.

Agenesis of the corpus callosum

This can be an isolated abnormality or may be associated with other major

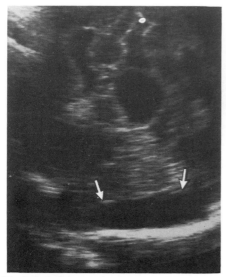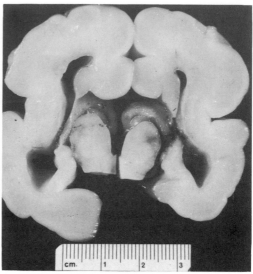

Fig. 8.8. *Left:* agenesis of corpus callosum, together with Dandy-Walker abnormality. The coronal plane shows abnormally shaped ventricles with a large and high third ventricle. There is an echo-free cystic area at the base of the posterior fossa *(arrowed)* representing a Dandy-Walker cyst. *Right:* autopsy specimen of brain with agenesis of corpus callosum.

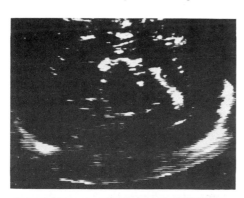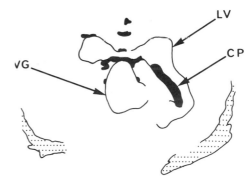

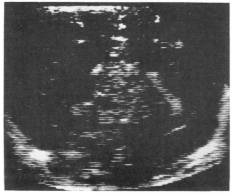

Fig. 8.9. Vein of Galen aneurysm. Coronal scans showing lateral ventricle (LV), choroid plexus (CP) and dilated vein of Galen (VG). Lower scan was made after 5ml of saline had been injected intravenously, and the previously echo-free vein of Galen filled with echoes from the dissolved gas in injected fluid. (Illustration by kind permission of Dr. Robert Jones and reproduced by courtesy of The Lancet.)

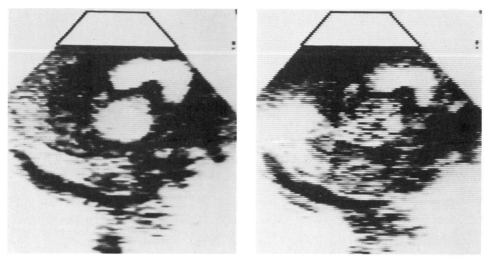

Fig. 8.10. Vein of Galen aneurysm. Sagittal scans showing an echo-free space *(left)* which fills with echoes following injection of intravenous saline *(right)*. This structure remained echogenic for 15 to 20 seconds after injection. (Posterior is to left in both scans.)

congenital abnormalities. Hydrocephalus may be present in some cases. The corpus callosum is normally an echo-free structure and easily recognised on ultrasound scans. The ultrasound appearance of agenesis of the corpus callosum is usually characteristic (Skeffington 1982). The lateral ventricles are widely separated and their shape is abnormal. The third ventricle is always situated high between the lateral ventricles. There is often dilatation of the posterior horns of the lateral ventricle particularly in a medial direction. Figures 8.7 and 8.8 illustrate examples of this condition. In addition, there are degrees of partial agenesis of the corpus callosum, which may be recognised on ultrasound scans.

Vein of Galen aneurysm

The vein of Galen is part of the venous sinus complex which drains blood from the brain. Only rarely is there an arteriovenous communication between one or more cerebral arteries and the vein of Galen, but this is an important cause of heart failure present at birth. It is often associated with other more extensive cerebral abnormalities. The infant may present at or shortly after birth with congestive cardiac failure and often cyanosis. Seizures and hydrocephalus also may be apparent. Long-term survival is rare.

The sonographic diagnosis is obvious and well described (Sauerbrei and Cooperberg 1981, Snider *et al.* 1981, Cubberley *et al.* 1982, Jones *et al.* 1982), but attention may be so strongly focused on the heart that a brain ultrasound scan is not considered. Trans-fontanelle images reveal a large echo-free space which represents the vein of Galen. This lies posterior to the third ventricle, and may extend asymmetrically across the midline. Communication of this echo-free cavity with the vascular system is confirmed by the injection of 1 to 2ml of saline intravenously.

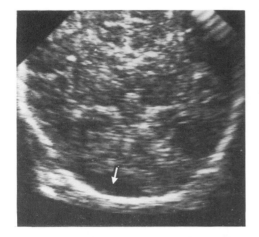

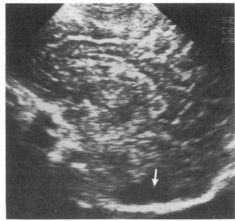

Fig. 8.11 *(above)*: cerebellar hypoplasia. The coronal *(left)* and sagittal *(right)* scans show an echo-free area in the region of left cerebellar hemisphere *(arrowed)*.

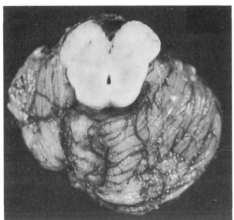

Fig. 8.12. *(left)*: cerebellar hypoplasia at autopsy. The scan of this case is illustrated in Figure 8.11 and shows hypoplasia isolated to left cerebellar hemisphere.

The dissolved micro-bubbles are clearly seen within the cavity for 10 to 15 seconds following the injection, and rapidly disappear as dilution in the circulation occurs (Figs. 8.9 and 8.10). Cubberley *et al.* (1982) also described the dilatation of the straight sinus which often communicates posteriorly with the aneurysm. Hydrocephalus may occur due to the mass effect of the aneurysm, as may other cerebral lesions related to the poor cerebral perfusion: *e.g.* periventricular leukomalacia, infarction and haemorrhage (Norman and Becker 1974).

Cerebellar malformations

Cerebellar agenesis is rare and hypoplasia occurs more commonly. The cerebellum gives a characteristic appearance on ultrasound examination, and abnormalities may be detected particularly on trans-fontanelle coronal scan directed into the posterior fossa. Cerebellar hypoplasia may also be associated with the Dandy-Walker abnormality. Hypoplasia may be asymmetrical, as shown in Figures 8.11 and 8.12.

REFERENCES

Adams, R. D., Sidman, R. L. (1968) *Introduction to Neuropathology.* New York: McGraw-Hill.

Cubberley, D. A., Jaffe, R. B., Nixon, G. W. (1982) 'Sonographic demonstration of Galenic arteriovenous malformations in the neonate.' *American Journal of Neuroradiology,* **3,** 435-439.

Jones, R. W. A., Allan, L. D., Tynan, M. J., Joseph, M. C. (1982) 'Ultrasound diagnosis of cerebral arteriovenous malformations in the newborn.' *Lancet,* **1,** 102-103.

Menkes, J. H. (1974) *Textbook of Child Neurology,* Philadelphia: Lea and Febiger.

Norman, M., Becker, L. (1974) 'Cerebral damage in neonates resulting from arteriovenous malformations of the vein of Galen.' *Journal of Neurology, Neurosurgery and Psychiatry,* **37,** 252-258.

Sauerbrei, E. E., Cooperberg, P. L. (1981) 'Neonatal brain: sonography of congenital abnormalities.' *American Journal of Roentgenology,* **136,** 1167-1170.

Skeffington, F. S. (1982) 'Agenesis of the corpus callosum: neonatal ultrasound appearances.' *Archives of Disease in Childhood,* **57,** 713-714.

Snider, A. R., Soifer, S. J., Silverman, N. H. (1981) 'Detection of intracranial arteriovenous fistula by two-dimensional ultrasonography.' *Circulation,* **63,** 1179-1185.

9
INFECTION

Infection may occur at various sites throughout the central nervous system, and ultrasound may contribute to diagnosis and management of some of these conditions. The infection is usually of viral or bacterial origin, and may be acquired before or after birth. Intra-uterine and postnatal infection will be discussed separately.

Intra-uterine infection
Neuropathological studies have distinguished different responses to infection. These may be inflammatory and destructive, or cause impairment of organ development with subsequent malformation.

Rubella
Cerebral lesions consist of a chronic meningeal reaction, with infiltration by inflammatory cells into the leptomeninges and perivascular spaces. Small areas of necrosis are found in the parenchyma, and are due to vasculitis with calcification. Subependymal pseudocysts have also been identified (Rorke and Spiro 1967, Shackleford *et al.* 1983). There is no known relationship between rubella and cerebral malformations. One infant with congenital rubella syndrome also presented with growth retardation, abnormal neurological findings, deafness, and

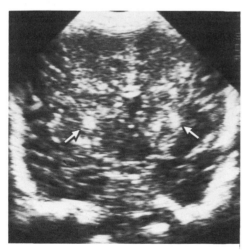

Fig. 9.1. Congenital rubella. Coronal scan through middle cranial fossa showing focal echogenic areas in thalamus *(arrowed)* together with periventricular echogenicity. Infant was born at term to woman who had contracted rubella in first trimester.

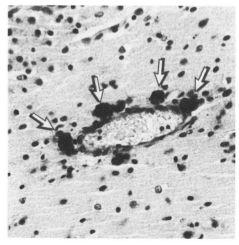

Fig. 9.2. Histological section from thalamus of infant with rubella embryopathy, showing areas of microcalcification *(arrowed)* surrounding small vessel.

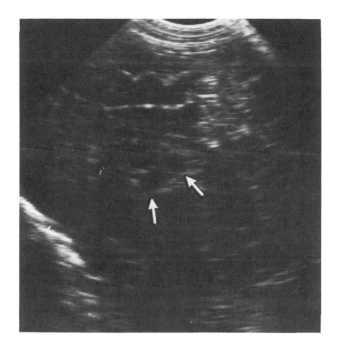

Fig. 9.3. Parasagittal scan showing multiple subependymal pseudocysts in term infant with proven congenital cytomegalovirus infection.

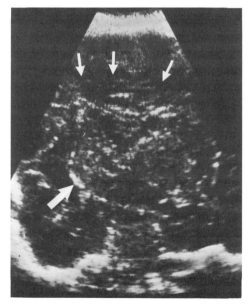 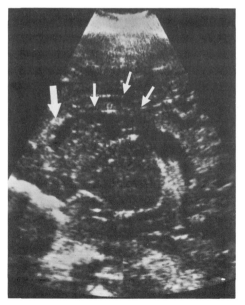

Fig. 9.4. Cytomegalovirus infection. Coronal *(left)* and parasagittal *(right)* views showing focal echogenic areas (probably calcification, *arrowed*) in periventricular white matter. In addition there are small areas of reduced echodensity *(small arrows)*.

111

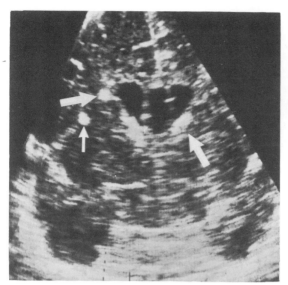

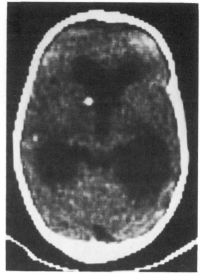

Fig. 9.5. Congenital toxoplasma infection. Coronal scan showing areas of periventricular echogenicity *(arrowed)* as well as discrete areas of increased echoes in region of thalamus *(small arrows)*. These are due to calcification.

Fig. 9.6. Computerised X-ray scan showing area of high attenuation in region of basal nuclei, consistent with calcification (same infant as in Figure 9.5).

patent ductus arteriosus. Ultrasound scans showed focal areas of increased echogenicity in the basal ganglia, compatible with calcification (Fig. 9.1). Post-mortem examination confirmed the presence of calcifications within the basal ganglia (Fig. 9.2).

Cytomegalovirus

Haymaker *et al.* (1954) described the cerebral lesions resulting from congenital cytomegalovirus (CMV) infection, and emphasized the preferential distribution within the olfactory bulb and walls of the lateral ventricles. This specific pattern of damage is attributed to a predilection of the virus for the subependymal plate (Shackleford *et al.* 1954, Haymaker *et al.* 1983). Lesions may also be present in the periventricular white matter, cortex, cerebellum, brainstem and spinal cord. The extent and size of the lesions are variable. Several authors have reported the association of CMV and cerebral malformations such as polymicrogyria and porencephalic cysts (Crome and France 1959, Navin and Angevine 1968).

The ultrasound appearances are variable. Multiple subependymal pseudocysts may be the only findings (Fig. 9.3) but calcification, focal areas of periventricular echodensity, and mild ventricular dilatation have all been observed (Fig. 9.4).

Toxoplasmosis

Intracerebral toxoplasma infection consists of a chronic focal meningo-encephalitis with necrosis, capillary proliferation, astrocytic reaction and inflammatory cell infiltration. Calcification occurs frequently. The necrotic foci often resolve into

TABLE 9.1
The ultrasound findings in six infants with intra-uterine viral infection

Aetiology	n	Basal ganglia calcifications	Periventricular white matter abnormalities	Ventricular dilatation
Rubella	1	Bilateral and extensive	No	No
Cytomegalo-virus	3	Minor calcification in one Two subependymal cysts	Small periventricular cysts in one	Mild in one only
Toxoplasmosis	1	Minor	Diffusely abnormal	Moderate

cystic lesions. Toxoplasmosis may be associated with cerebral malformations or hydranenephaly (Crome and Sylvester 1958, Altshuler 1973). Ultrasound scanning may show markedly increased echodensity within the periventricular white matter, probably due to microcalcifications (Figs. 9.5 and 9.6). Nodular ependymitis with subsequent stenosis of the aqueduct of Sylvius has been described, and hydro-cephalus is a frequent complication of this condition. The ultrasound findings in five cases of intra-uterine infection are summarised in Table 9.1. Other infective agents such as syphilis, herpes simplex and candida have been reported to cause cerebral damage, but we have not seen examples of these.

Meningitis

The ultrasound findings in infants with complicated meningitis have been reported by Edwards *et al.* (1982). They found the earliest ultrasound abnormality to be a focal increase in the echodensity of the cerebral cortex. It was thought to be due to meningo-encephalitis, which they recognised in six of 20 infants. Echodensity was seen predominantly in the cortical grey matter and caused accentuation of the

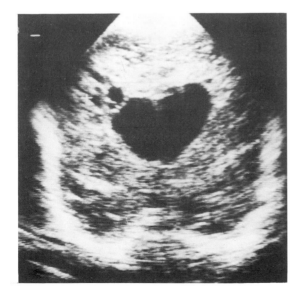

Fig. 9.7. Acute haemophilus meningitis. Coronal scan showing a widespread increase in echoes throughout the brain together with ventricular dilatation and periventricular cyst formation.

TABLE 9.2
Details of 10 infants with neonatal bacterial meningitis

Meningitis	n	Parenchymal lesions	Extracerebral space enlargement	Ventricular dilatation
Listeriosis	3	—	—	—
Streptococcus B Group	2	—	+ (in one only)	—
Proteus	1	Multiple peri-ventricular cysts	—	Required shunting
Proteus	1	Temporo-occipital abscess	—	Required shunting
Haemophilus	2	Right frontal abscess. Multiple cystic degeneration	+ (in one only)	Progressive in both cases
Pneumococcus	1	Basal ganglia echodensity	+	—
Unknown organism	1	—	—	Thrombi with transient dilatation

grey/white matter interface. In some patients this appearance was deeper in the brain, and was possibly due to early abscess formation. These areas resolved with antibiotic therapy. Infants with meningitis may develop more widespread echodensity throughout the brain (Reeder and Sanders 1983), obscuring anatomical landmarks. This diffuse change is thought to represent oedema (Fig. 9.7).

The virulence of the organism producing meningitis is likely to influence the ultrasound appearances. We have seen 11 infants with bacterial meningitis (Table 9.2). Three infants with Listeria monocytogenes meningitis, and two with Group B beta haemolytic streptococcus meningitis, showed no abnormalities on ultrasound examination. The most extensive ultrasound abnormalities were seen in infants with meningitis due to proteus and haemophilus infections. Major abnormalities were found in the periventricular white matter, but these infants were not scanned in the acute stages of their illness. Multiple periventricular cysts were seen in two cases, three to six weeks after the onset of infection (Fig. 9.8). One infant with proteus meningitis developed a large temporo-occipital abscess (Fig. 9.9). Four infants developed ventricular dilatation.

Ventricular bands, membranes and septi have been reported in the presence of ventriculitis (Hill et al. 1981, Edwards et al. 1982, Reeder and Sanders 1983). In some cases these occur early in the acute stages of the infection, and in other patients during the convalescent phase of the illness. These are probably due to arachnoid adhesions or inflammatory exudate, and are usually seen once ventricular dilatation has occurred. Figure 9.10 shows an example of this appearance.

Ventriculomegaly is commonly seen following meningitis, and is usually due to inflammatory exudate causing obstruction to the passage of cerebrospinal fluid at the base of the skull. Acquired obstructions may also occur in the aqueduct of Sylvius. In one study, ventricular dilatation occurred in 60 per cent of infants examined by ultrasound following meningitis (Edwards et al. 1982). Others have

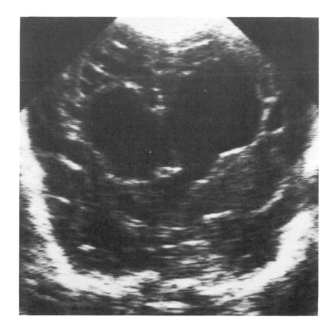

Fig. 9.8. Coronal scan six weeks after proteus meningitis. There are multiple periventricular cysts together with marked ventricular dilatation.

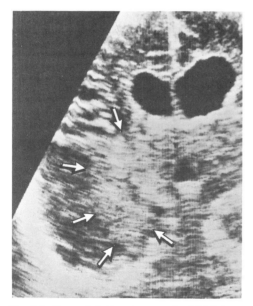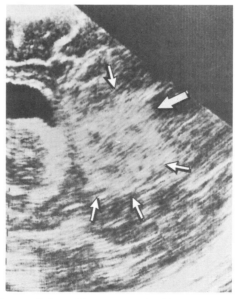

Fig. 9.9. Coronal *(left)* and parasagittal *(right)* scans from an infant with proteus meningitis. There is an area of intense echogenicity *(arrows)* in temporo-occipital region of brain corresponding to abscess formation.

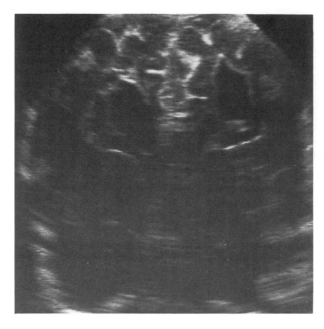

Fig. 9.10. Scan from an infant with Staph. Epidermidis meningitis following ventricular shunt insertion. There are echogenic bands lying within ventricles. Cerebral atrophy is also present.

confirmed these findings (Hill *et al.* 1981, Reeder and Sanders 1983). Asymmetrical ventricular dilatation may occur following meningitis and is probably due to focal areas of cerebral atrophy. Subependymal pseudocyst formation has also been reported following ventriculitis.

Abscess and cavitation are well recognised following meningo-encephalitis (Hill *et al.* 1981, Edwards *et al.* 1982). Edwards *et al.* reported discrete areas of dense echoes of both frontal lobes in one infant. Three days later the scan showed progressive reduction in the echodensity, with eventual central echo-lucency believed to be an abscess cavity. This infant had proteus Mirabilis sepsis (Fig. 9.9).

The ultrasound detection of cerebral abscess formation has occasionally been reported. Regular ultrasound scans were performed following experimental abscess formation in the brain of a dog, and a hyperechoic rim with a hypo-echoic centre was initially noted at three days (Enzmann *et al.* 1981). The edge of the lesion was well demarcated from the surrounding brain, which was of lower echodensity. Oedema surrounding the abscess, well seen by CT examination, was not obvious on ultrasound. With healing, two weeks following initiation of the lesion, the echodense rim increased in thickness and the central region of lower echodensity diminished in size. It is likely that in the infant, cerebral abscess can reliably be detected by ultrasound.

REFERENCES

Altshuler, G. (1973) 'Toxoplasmosis as a cause of hydranencephaly.' *American Journal of Diseases in Children,* **125,** 251-252.
Crome, L., France, N. E. (1959) 'Microgyria and cytomegalic inclusion disease in infancy.' *Journal of Clinical Pathology,* **12,** 427-434.
Crome, L., Sylvester, P. E. (1958) 'Hydranencephaly (hydrencephaly).' *Archives of Disease in*

Childhood, **33,** 235-245.

Edwards, M. K., Brown, D. L., Chua, G. T. (1982) 'Complicated infantile meningitis: evaluation by real-time sonography.' *American Journal of Neuroradiology, 3,* 431-434.

Enzmann, D. R., Britt, R. H., Lyons, B., Carroll, B., Wilson, D. A., Buston, J. (1981) 'High resolution ultrasound evaluation of experimental brain abscess evolution: comparison with computer tomography and neuropathology.' *Radiology,* **142,** 95-102.

Haymaker, W., Girdany, B. R., Stephens, J. (1954) 'Cerebral involvement with advanced periventricular calcifications in generalised cytomegalic inclusion disease in the newborn.' *Journal of Neuropathology and Experimental Neurology,* **13,** 562-586.

Hill, A., Shackelford, G. D., Volpe, J. J. (1981) 'Ventriculitis with neonatal bacterial meningitis: identification by real-time ultrasound.' *Journal of Pediatrics,* **99,** 133-136.

Navin, M. J., Angevine, J. M. (1968) 'Congenital cytomegalic inclusion disease with porencephaly.' *Neurology,* **18,** 470-472.

Reeder, J. D., Sanders, R. C. (1983) 'Ventriculitis in the neonate: recognition by sonography.' *American Journal of Neuroradiology,* **4,** 37-41.

Rorke, L., Spiro, A. J. (1967) 'Cerebral lesions in congenital rubella syndrome.' *Journal of Pediatrics,* **70,** 243-255.

Shackelford, G. D., Fulling, K. H., Glasier, C. M. (1983) 'Cysts of the subependymal germinal matrix. Sonographic demonstration with pathologic correlation.' *Radiology,* **149,** 117-21.

10
MISCELLANEOUS ABNORMALITIES

Oedema

Reliable detection of cerebral oedema by ultrasound scanning is often quite difficult and CT is a much more sensitive imaging modality for this diagnosis. There are certain babies who have sustained hypoxic-ischaemic encephalopathy who do show abnormalities which are recognisable by ultrasound (Babcock and Ball 1983). In some cases following asphyxia there is a uniform increase in tissue echogenicity, obscuring anatomical features throughout the brain. This appearance has also been seen following symptomatic hypoglycaemia, heart failure, sepsis, renal failure, metabolic disorders and child abuse (Fig 10.1). Figure 10.2 is of an infant scanned at two weeks, following very severe asphyxia at birth. This scan shows markedly increased echodensity in the thalamus and cortical regions, in contrast to the periventricular areas. This appearance persisted for at least two weeks. We have failed to see similar appearances in apparently equally severely asphyxiated infants. We suggest that this is due to intracerebral vasogenic oedema opening up tissue spaces, thus causing a marked increase in echo interfaces.

Skeffington and Pearse (1983) have coined the phrase the 'bright brain' to describe the appearance of diffuse echogenicity. In 12 of 13 infants they described with this appearance, there was a clinical history suggestive of cerebral insult. Dampened vascular excursions can be identified by real-time ultrasound examination, and indicate a disturbance in bloodflow (Williams 1983). Focal or universal

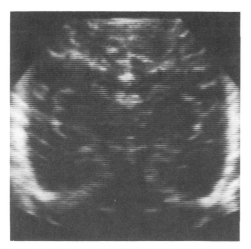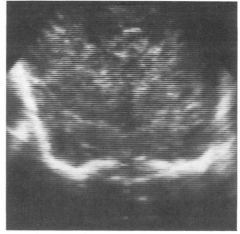

Fig. 10.1. Cerebral oedema. *Left:* early coronal scan from infant suffering from severe perinatal asphyxia. *Right:* scan from same infant some days later showing diffuse increase in echoes from parenchyma, with loss of normal landmarks. On real-time imaging there was marked loss of vascular pulsations.

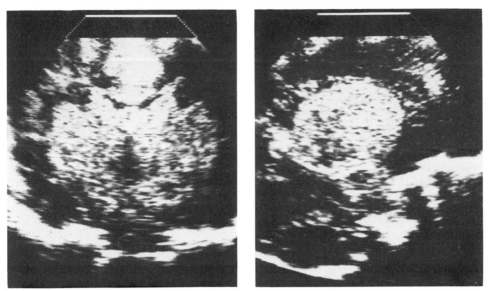

Fig. 10.2. Cerebral oedema in an infant scanned 10 days after sustaining severe perinatal asphyxia. Coronal scan *(above left)* shows marked echogenicity in region of basal nuclei and interhemispheric fissure. Ventricles, periventricular white matter and convexity cortex appear normal. Parasagittal scan *(above right)* shows thalamus to be extremely echogenic, and rest of brain is normal in appearance.

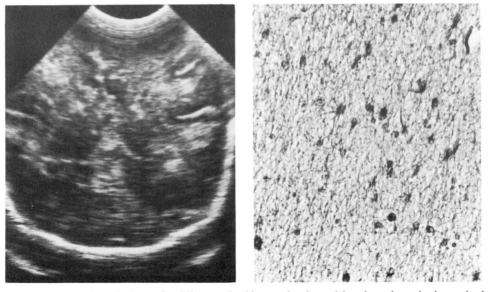

Fig. 10.3. Extensive gliosis. *Left:* diffuse and widespread echogenicity throughout both cerebral hemispheres, possibly sparing grey matter. *Right:* histology revealed extensive gliosis involving white matter.

119

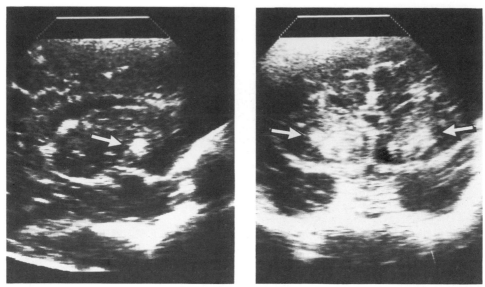

Fig. 10.4. Intrathalamic calcification. Scans from a developmentally retarded infant showing areas of marked echogenicity *(arrowed)* in thalamus on both coronal *(left)* and parasagittal *(right)* sections. Calcification was confirmed on CT scans.

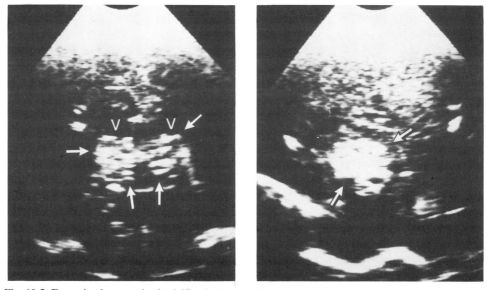

Fig. 10.5. Extensive intracerebral calcification in an infant with Fahr's syndrome. Massive intrathalamic echodense areas *(arrowed)* seen on coronal *(left)* and parasagittal scans *(right)*. The calcium was seen on a plain skull X-ray. (V = lateral ventricle).

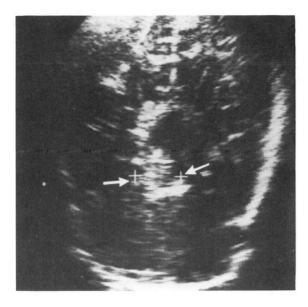

Fig. 10.6. Medulloblastoma. Coronal scan showing an irregular echogenic area in posterior fossa *(arrowed)*. This was shown to be a medulloblastoma on biopsy.

decrease in intracranial vascular pulsations are often associated with the appearance of oedema. Diffuse echogenicity throughout the brain may however not be due to oedema and diagnosis may be uncertain. In one case of perinatal asphyxia in a full-term infant, ultrasound scans showed diffusely increased echodensity involving the entire white matter. At post-mortem extensive gliosis was seen corresponding to the areas of density seen on the ultrasound scans. (Fig. 10.3).

Calcification

Intracranial calcification may occur in the newborn due to a number of different conditions including infection, asphyxia and tumour. The detection of calcification depends on its position and density. Dykes *et al.* (1982) described five infants who showed intracranial calcification detected by ultrasound. All had periventricular calcification without acoustic shadowing and all had proven or strongly suspected prenatal toxoplasmosis or cytomegalovirus infection. Computerised tomography confirmed the periventricular calcification in all cases. Periventricular intracranial calcification has also been detected by Sauerbrei and Cooperberg (1981). Computerised tomography is five to 15 times more sensitive than a plain x-ray in the detection of intracranial calcification (Norman *et al.* 1978), but ultrasound may be even more sensitive than CT in the newborn brain.

Focal intrathalamic calcification following asphyxic injury, rubella or from unknown causation has been identified. The appearances in these infants were remarkably uniform (Figs. 10.4 and 10.5). Small discrete areas of echodensity appeared bilaterally within the midpart of the thalamus and were seen on both coronal and parasagittal images. At post-mortem, microcalcification was present in the thalamus corresponding exactly in position to the echoes seen on ultrasound. In one of these infants the calcification was not seen on a CT examination.

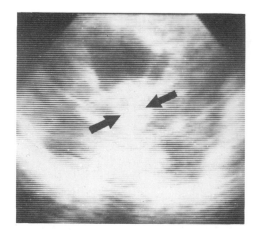

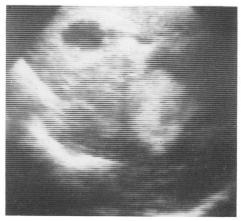

Fig. 10.7. Pinealoblastoma. A midline echogenic mass *(arrows)* is seen on coronal section *(above left)*, and on parasagittal section *(above right)* is seen to be situated posterior to third ventricle.

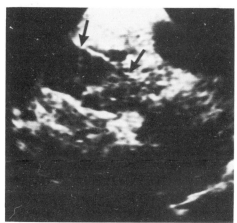

Fig. 10.8 *(left):* congenital brain tumour. A massive echogenic tumour *(arrowed)* is present on parasagittal section. This is associated with multiple echo-free cystic cavities. This was found to be a primitive neuronal tumour on biopsy. (Posterior is to left of scan. We are grateful to Dr. Rosemary Shannon for allowing us to study her patient.)

Tumour

There have been a number of case reports of congenital tumours detected by ultrasound examination (Heimburger *et al.* 1978, Babcock and Han 1981, Horbar *et al.* 1982). These include choroid plexus angioma, ependymoma, astrocytoma, teratoma and pineal tumour. The latter appeared to be cystic (Heimburger *et al.* 1978), and the teratoma (Horbar *et al.* 1982) was associated with hydrocephalus. The ultrasound scan showed large and small cystic spaces within the tumour tissue. The astrocytomas affected the optic chiasm in one infant and the thalamus in another (Babcock and Han 1981). These tumours were echodense, were associated with some distortion of normal anatomy, together with ventricular dilatation in one and a loculated fluid collection in another. We have seen one infant with a medulloblastoma arising from the brainstem who had associated hydrocephalus. The tumour was echodense and had an irregular outline (Fig. 10.6) and was observed to reduce in size with radiotherapy. The tumour response to radiation therapy can be readily monitored by ultrasound. Tumour may be present in an

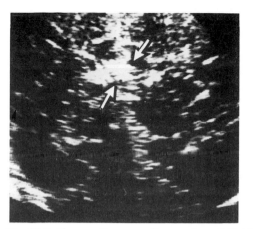
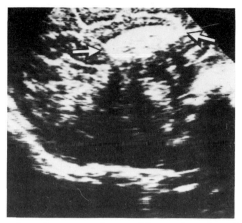

Fig. 10.9. Lipoma of corpus callosum. A small highly echogenic structure *(arrowed)* is seen in region of corpus callosum on coronal scan *(left)* and sagittal scan *(right)*.

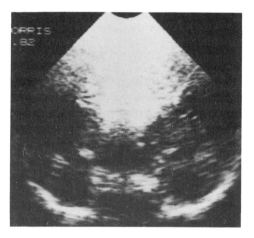
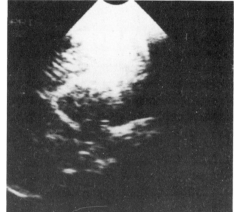

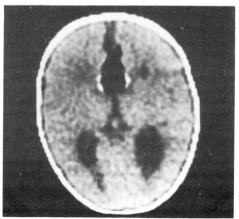

Fig. 10.10. Massive intracerebral lipoma. Scans from infant presenting at birth with a soft swelling in middle of forehead. Ultrasound showed on coronal scan *(above left)* an intensely echogenic mass penetrating through skull and infiltrating between cerebral hemispheres. On sagittal scan *(above right)* anterior (right) and posterior (left) extent of this lipomatous mass can be seen. *Left:* computerised X-ray scan of same infant. Anteriorly placed midline lipoma is radiolucent on CT in contrast to its marked echodensity on ultrasound examination. (We are grateful to Dr. John Moore for allowing us to study his patient.)

123

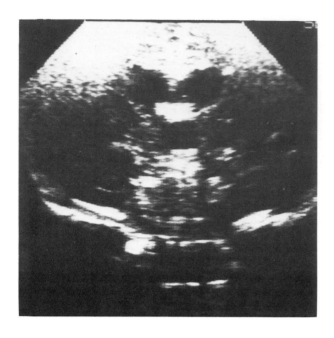

Fig. 10.11. Cerebral atrophy. Dilated lateral ventricles and third ventricles together with separation of interhemispheric fissure. Severe atrophy was confirmed at autopsy.

infant presenting with hydrocephalus of obscure cause but it is a rare condition in the first few months of life (Figs. 10.7 and 10.8). Ultrasound is not yet sufficiently reliable to exclude a tumour causing hydrocephalus and CT should be complementary to it.

Lipoma

A lipomatous malformation is a well-recognised midline abnormality of the central nervous system and the most likely site within the brain is the corpus callosum. A lipoma appears as an intensely echodense area within the corpus callosum (Fig. 10.9) present from birth, and should not be confused with haemorrhage. On CT examination this abnormality is of low attenuation (Sauerbrei and Cooperberg 1981). In one infant a fluctuant midline lipomatous swelling was present on the forehead. Intracranial ultrasound scans revealed a large echodense midline lipomatous malformation involving much of the frontal lobe (Fig. 10.10). Lipomata may also occur in the spine.

Cerebral atrophy

Cerebral atrophy is due to destruction of brain tissue and may be due to a variety of perinatal insults. The atrophy may be global, leaving a shrunken brain with damage to the basal nuclei. Mature infants sustaining hypoxic-ischaemic injury are more likely to sustain damage to the cerebral mantle with resulting contraction of the brain and widening of the Sylvian fissures together with marked separation of the interhemispheric fissure in the midline. In addition cortical cystic degeneration may occur separately or in conjunction with these other features.

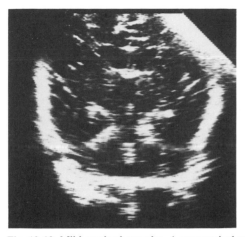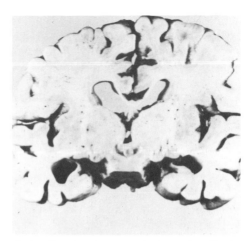

Fig. 10.12. Mild cerebral atrophy. Asymmetrical ventricular dilatation due to cerebral atrophy affecting mainly left periventricular white matter and basal nuclei. There is compensatory ventricular dilatation particularly on left side.

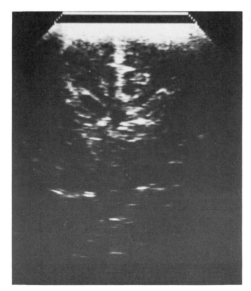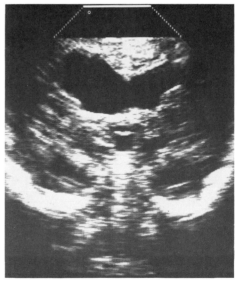

Fig. 10.13. Univentricular dilatation. Coronal scan from infant with persistent univentricular dilatation of the lateral ventricle. Haemorrhage was never detected, and this appearance persisted from birth until he was last scanned at six months of age.

Fig. 10.14. Cerebral atrophy and post-haemorrhagic ventricular dilatation. Persistent and asymmetrical dilatation of lateral ventricles as well as enlargement of the third ventricle. This infant was known to have had intraventricular haemorrhage in newborn period.

In the past the term 'hydrocephalus *ex vacuo*' was used to describe cerebral atrophy. This term referred to the ventricular dilatation that occurs in response to cerebral damage and parenchymal volume loss. As atrophy is usually a non-uniform process, ventricular dilatation may be irregular and asymmetrical and may include the third ventricle (Fig. 10.11). Ischaemia or hypoxia in the premature infant may cause periventricular leukomalacia with subsequent cyst formation as described in Chapter 6. These insults may also lead to damage in basal nuclei with asymmetrical ventricular dilatation (Fig. 10.12). This appearance of asymmetrical ventricular dilatation is not uncommon in surviving infants. These changes occur within weeks of the cerebral insult, and are persistent. Sometimes only one ventricle is involved (Fig. 10.13). The shapes of the ventricles are not distended or ballooned as occurs in post-haemorrhagic ventricular dilatation, but are more irregular and squat in outline. Asymmetrical ventricular dilatation is a common finding during the acute phase of germinal matrix haemorrhage when liquid blood distends one ventricle. It is important not to confuse cerebral atrophy with this condition which usually resolves within several weeks. Atrophy does not resolve with time. It is therefore inadvisable to diagnose atrophy in the presence of intraventricular haemorrhage.

Inevitably one will scan an infant who shows marked ventricular dilatation together with a considerable degree of asymmetry (Fig. 10.14). It may be impossible to determine if post-haemorrhagic ventricular dilatation or atrophy is present or if there is a combination of the two processes. Examination of the head growth may not be a reliable contributory investigation, although in infants who have sustained the most severe degrees of cerebral atrophy the head usually fails to grow. Less severe degrees of atrophy occur in the presence of normal increases in head size. There is no good imaging modality that will identify all degrees of cerebral atrophy, and confusion between ventricular dilatation and atrophy will inevitably exist.

REFERENCES

Babcock, D. S., Han, B. K. (1981) 'The accuracy of high resolution, real-time ultrasonography of the head in infancy.' *Radiology*, **139**, 665-676.
—— Ball, W. (1983) 'Postasphyxial encephalopathy in full-term infants: ultrasound diagnosis.' *Radiology*, **148**, 417-423.
Dykes, F. D., Ahmann, P. A., Lazzara, A. (1982) 'Cranial ultrasound in the detection of intracranial calcification.' *Journal of Pediatrics*, **100**, 404-408.
Heimburger, R. F., Fry, F. J., Patrick, J. T., Gardner, G., Gresham, E. (1978) 'Ultrasound brain tomography for infants and young children.' *Perinatology Neonatology*, **2**, 27-31.
Horbar, J. D., Leahy, K., Lucey, J. F. (1982) 'Real-time ultrasonography. Its use in diagnoses and management of neonatal hydrocephalus.' *American Journal of Diseases in Children*, **136**, 693-696.
Norman, D., Diamond, C., Boyd, D. (1978) 'Relative detectability of intracranial calcifications on computed tomography and skull radiography.' *Journal of Computer Assisted Tomography*, **2**, 61-64.
Sauerbrei, E. E., Cooperberg, P. L. (1981) 'Neonatal brain: sonography of congenital abnormalities.' *American Journal of Radiology*, **136**, 1167-1170.
Skeffington, F. S., Pearse, R. G. (1983) 'The "bright brain".' *Archives of Disease in Childhood*, **58**, 509-511.
Williams, J. L. (1983) 'Intracranial vascular pulsations in pediatric neurosonology.' *Journal of Ultrasound in Medicine*, **2**, 485-488.

11
HYDROCEPHALUS AND VENTRICULAR SHUNTS

Hydrocephalus

Production of cerebrospinal fluid (CSF) takes place predominantly in the choroid plexus of the lateral ventricles. The fluid flows downward through the foramen of Monro, into the third ventricle, passes through the aqueduct of Sylvius and enters the fourth ventricle. Passage through the foramina of Luschka and Magendie delivers the CSF into the spinal canal and basilar cisterns. CSF flows upward over the convexities of the hemispheres to the arachnoid villi, and from there absorption into the superior sagittal sinus occurs. Normally, only 15 per cent or less of the CSF is reabsorbed by alternate pathways, such as the ependyma, perineural spaces, or back through the choroid plexus.

Hydrocephalus is a descriptive term referring to a clinical appearance that may include a large head, bulging fontanelles, dilated scalp veins, 'sunsetting' of the eyes or lethargy with vomiting. In pathological states, excessive CSF accumulates within the bony vault. Overproduction of CSF by a choroid plexus papilloma may deliver large enough quantities of CSF to the system to exceed the reabsorptive capabilities. Conversely, any obstruction along the pathway produces proximal distension. If the obstruction occurs anywhere within the ventricular system (from the foramen of Monro to the foramina of Luschka and Magendie), the process is referred to as intraventricular obstructive hydrocephalus (IVOH) or non-communicating hydrocephalus (Figs. 11.1 to 11.3). If the block occurs within the pathway from the basilar cisterns to the arachnoid villi, it is called an extraventricular obstructive hydrocephalus (EVOH) or communicating hydrocephalus (Figs. 11.4 and 11.5). Table 11.1 summarizes the causes of these two types.

TABLE 11.1

Causes of congenital hydrocephalus based on whether or not there is communication with the extracranial CSF space

Non-communicating *IVOH*	Communicating *EVOH*
Aqueduct stenosis	Extra-axial arachnoid cyst
Arnold-Chiari malformation	Idiopathic
Dandy-Walker syndrome	Secondary—haemorrhage
Vein of Galen aneurysm	or inflammation

External hydrocephalus is a term used to describe a predominant excess of CSF in the subarachnoid space with relatively little if any increase in the volume of the intracerebral ventricles. It may be due to a developmental abnormality of the arachnoid granulations, or may follow haemorrhage. This condition is not uncommonly seen on ultrasound scans, and about 5 per cent of infants referred for

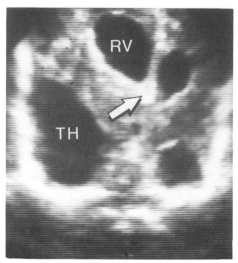

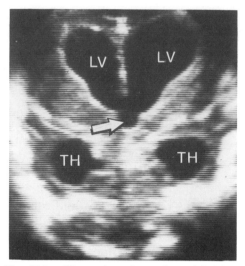

Fig. 11.1. Right foramen of Monro obstruction. Coronal sonogram demonstrates greater enlargement of right ventricle (RV) and temporal horn (TH) than on left side. A clot was found occluding foramen of Monro *(arrow)*.

Fig. 11.2a. Obstruction of aqueduct of Sylvius. Coronal sonogram shows enlargement of both lateral ventricles (LV) and temporal horns (TH). Widely patent foramen of Monro *(arrow)* is present on each side and leads to prominent third ventricle.

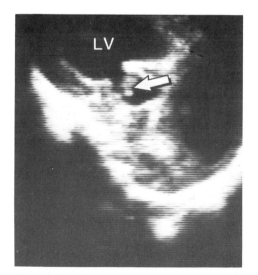

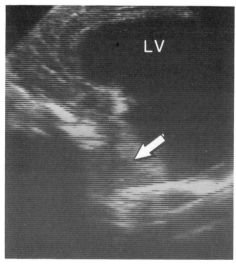

Fig. 11.2b. Obstruction of the aqueduct of Sylvius. Parasagittal sonogram illustrates enlarged lateral ventricle (LV), wide foramen of Monro and prominent massa intermedia *(arrow)* within dilated third ventricle. Fourth ventricle is normal. Here obstruction was due to gliosis within aqueduct from a previous intraventricular haemorrhage.

Fig. 11.3. Arnold-Chiari II malformation. Sagittal sonogram shows enlarged lateral ventricle (LV) and relatively prominent massa intermedia within a dysmorphic third ventricle. There is caudal displacement of fastigium *(arrow)* of fourth ventricle. A meningocele was present in lumbar spine of this patient.

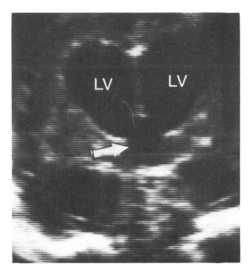

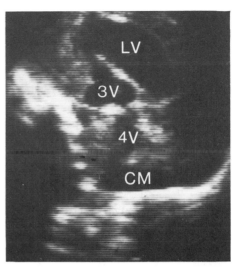

Fig. 11.4. Communicating hydrocephalus (EVOH). The coronal sonogram shows dilated lateral ventricles (LV) and large third ventricle *(arrow)*. Fourth ventricle is not seen in this projection.

Fig. 11.5. Communicating hydrocephalus (EVOH). The sagittal sonogram illustrates widely patent lateral (LV), third (3V) and fourth (4V) ventricles. Cisterna magna (CM) is also large. A previous intracranial haemorrhage in this patient resulted in meningeal thickening over convexities and partial obstruction of CSF return through arachnoid granulations.

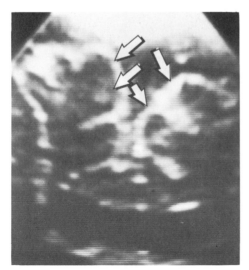

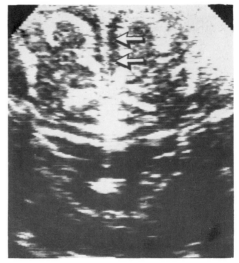

Fig. 11.6. Excessive CSF in interhemispheric fissure. A magnified coronal sonogram demonstrates excessive extra-axial CSF separating two cortical layers *(arrows)* in interhemispheric fissure.

Fig. 11.7. External hydrocephalus. This coronal scan clearly shows falx *(arrowed)* within widened interhemispheric fissure. Surface of brain is also apparent. There is an excess of subarachnoid CSF without ventricular dilatation. (Reproduced by permission of the editor of the British Journal of Radiology.)

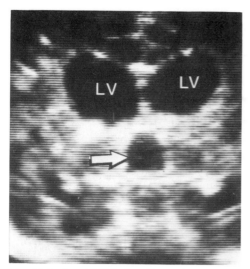 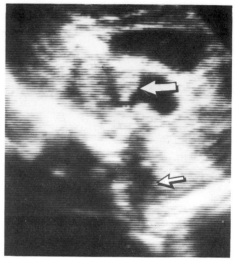

Fig. 11.8. Arnold-Chiari malformation. Coronal sonogram demonstrating bilateral lateral ventricular enlargement (LV) and prominent third ventricle *(arrow)*. The posterior fossa is not clearly seen in the section.

Fig. 11.9. Arnold-Chiari malformation. Sagittal sonogram shows prominent massa intermedia *(top arrow)* within enlarged third ventricle. Caudal displacement of large fourth ventricle is shown by inferior displacement of fastigium *(bottom arrow)*.

scanning because of a large head have this abnormality. It is characterized by normal lateral ventricles together with visualization of the surface of the brain. The gyri and sulci are very prominent because of excessive subarachnoid fluid (Figs. 11.6 and 11.7). A stand-off water path may help in the detection of this condition, but it may not be possible to distinguish it confidently from cerebral atrophy, subarachnoid haemorrhage or EVOH. Hydrocephalus *ex vacuo* refers to the enlargement of the ventricular spaces due to destruction of cerebral tissue. This term is misleading, and cerebral atrophy is more appropriate.

Mass lesions such as tumours or arachnoid cysts may produce delayed IVOH by their location along the ventricular system. Congenital obstructive lesions, such as aqueductal stenosis (Figs. 11.2 and 11.3), Arnold-Chiari malformation (Figs. 11.8 and 11.9), achondroplasia, and Dandy-Walker syndrome (Figs. 7.6 to 7.8) usually produce more immediate IVOH. Haemorrhage or infection producing aqueductal or foraminal stenosis is far more common (Scotti *et al.* 1980). Post-inflammatory thickening (haemorrhage or infection) of the meninges and the arachnoid villi accounts for almost all of the cases of EVOH (see Chapters 5 and 9). Arteriovenous malformations and meningeal spread of tumour are more unlikely causes.

Follow-up examinations are important adjuncts to the clinical evaluation of the infant or young child who is at risk for ventricular enlargement (Babcock and Han 1980, Yamada *et al.* 1982). Increasing size of the ventricles or progressive rounding of the ventricular angles indicates worsening hydrocephalus. Increasing fluid accumulation in the cisterna magna, basilar cisterns, Sylvian fissures and interhemispheric fissure are supporting features.

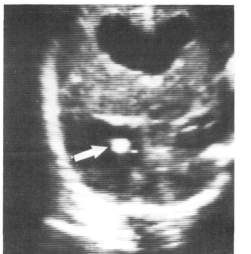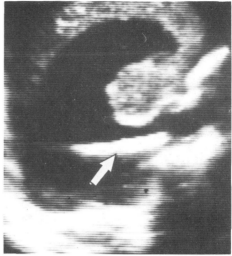

Fig. 11.10. Ventricular shunt tube placement. Coronal sonogram reveals strongly reflective catheter *(arrow)* within temporal horn of right lateral ventricle. Note equally echogenic choroid just above the shunt tube. *Right:* Parasagittal sonogram demonstrates echogenic catheter *(arrow)* within temporal horn. The close proximity of choroid increases the chance of occlusion. (Posterior is to left of scan.)

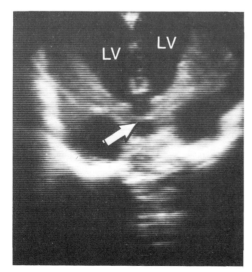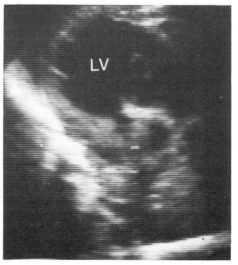

Fig. 11.11. Slit ventricle syndrome. *Left:* pre-shunt coronal sonogram shows marked dilatation of lateral (LV) and third ventricles. The crossing massa intermedia *(arrow)* is well seen. *Right:* sagittal sonogram shows marked enlargement of lateral ventricle (LV) and prominence of third and fourth ventricles. Patient had suffered a previous intracranial haemorrhage.

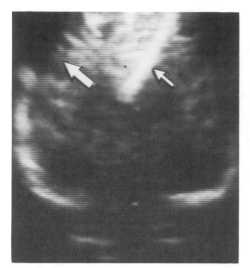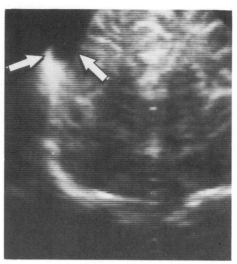

Fig. 11.12. Slit ventricle syndrome. *Left:* following placement of ventriculo-peritoneal shunt *(right arrow)*, rapid decompression occurred and enlarged ventricles are no longer seen. Note separation of cortex and inner table over right convexity *(left arrow)* due to fluid accumulation. *Right:* echogenic shunt tube has been removed and a repeat coronal sonogram demonstrates slight progression of subdural fluid accumulations *(arrows)*.

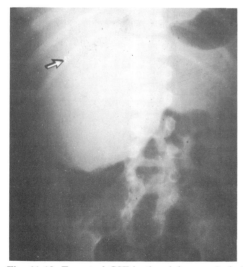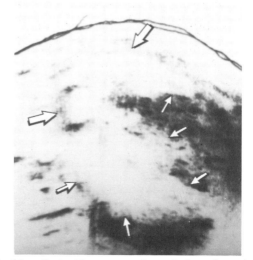

Fig. 11.13. Encysted CSF in the abdomen. *Left:* in this patient with a suspected ventriculo-peritoneal shunt malfunction, a plain film of abdomen demonstrates a soft tissue mass in right upper quadrant. Opaque tip of shunt tube *(arrow)* is located in the mass. *Right:* longitudinal B-scan of abdomen shows multiple fluid collections *(arrows)* in peritoneal space. These closed collections of CSF have obstructed drainage of ventriculo-peritoneal shunt.

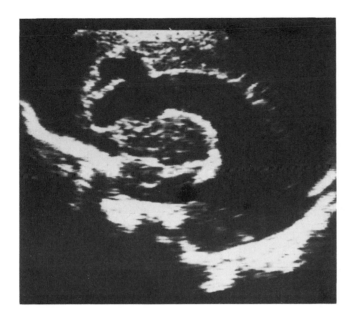

Fig. 11.14. Cystic degeneration in a needle track. This infant had multiple attempts to blindly needle the lateral ventricle. Supraventricular cyst in communication with lateral ventricle developed seven days after last attempt.

Ventricular shunts

When the decision to shunt is made, intra-operative guidance may aid the neurosurgical team in the placement of the catheter tip in the anterior horn of the appropriate lateral ventricle (Fig. 11.10) (Shkolnik 1981, 1982; Chandler *et al.* 1982; Knake *et al.* 1982). There is no choroid plexus anterior to the foramen of Monro, so that choroid plugging of the perforations at the tube tip is avoided.

Serial ultrasound examination following ventricular shunting procedures is important to identify adequate shunt functioning. Decompression is indicated by a decrease in the size of the ventricles, more acute angles at the ventricular margins, and increasing mantle thickening. Fracture or disconnection of extraventricular tubing can best be identified by radiographic means.

Occasionally, decompression of the enlarged ventricles occurs too rapidly, with tearing of the bridging cortical veins and subdural haematoma formation (Chapter 3). Such high convexity lesions can best be demonstrated when a water-path device is used. A water-filled latex examination glove works quite well. Overdrainage of enlarged ventricles may also result in the development of the 'slit ventricle syndrome' (Figs. 11.11 and 11.12) (Hyde-Rowan *et al.* 1982). The placement of high-resistance anti-syphon devices in line with the reservoir system will prevent the too rapid decompression of the ventricular system. Many different subcutaneous reservoirs and valve devices are available. On/off switches allow for encouragement of alternative pathways for CSF reabsorption. Occluders in the system permit patency evaluation at either end of the system. Access reservoirs permit aspiration of CSF for laboratory analysis and culture. Variable resistance shunts can also be placed to prevent rapid decompression. Some manufacturers have placed these different devices in tandem to permit the subcutaneous 'valve' to

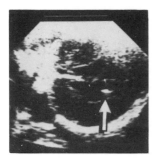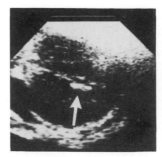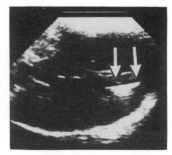

Fig. 11.15. Ultrasound-guided needle placement. Three coronal scans made by placing transducer on temporoparietal bone. The echodense needle *(arrowed)* can be seen progressively penetrating cerebrum through fontanelle, and is advanced under ultrasound guidance to lie within mid-portion of lateral ventricle (Levene 1982.) (Reproduced by permission of the editor of the British Medical Journal.)

perform several functions.

The distal end of the shunt tubing can be placed in the gall bladder, pleural space, mediastinal veins or peritoneal space. The peritoneal cavity is most commonly used. If the CSF causes peritoneal irritation, the omentum may wall off the tip of the tube (Agha *et al.* 1983). Such distal tube CSF collections may be unilocular or multilocular, and are easily identified with abdominal ultrasound (Fig. 11.13).

Occasionally it may be necessary to aspirate CSF or to instil antibiotics directly into the lateral ventricle. Blind placement of a needle through the anterior fontanelle may cause cystic degeneration of the supraventricular parenchyma (Fig. 11.14). Placement of a needle into the latcral ventricle is possible under real-time ultrasound control. The transducer can be placed over the parietal region to obtain a coronal image. Entry of the needle is then seen as it passes into and through the brain. The direction of the needle can be controlled and the location of the tip within the body of the ventricle assured (Fig. 11.15) (Levene 1982).

REFERENCES

Agha, F. P., Amendola, M. A., Shirazi, K. K., Amendola, B. E., Chandler, W. F. (1983) 'Unusual abdominal complications of ventriculoperitoneal shunts.' *Radiology,* **146,** 323-326.
Babcock, D. S., Han, B. K. (1980) 'Cranial sonographic findings in meningomyelocele.' *American Journal of Roentgenology,* **136,** 563-568 (see also: *American Journal of Neuroradiology,* **1,** 493-499).
Chandler, W. F., Knake, J. E., McGillicuddy, J. E., Lillehei, K. O., Silver, T. E. (1982) 'Intraoperative use of real-time ultrasonography in neurosurgery.' *Journal of Neurosurgery,* **57,** 157-163.
Hyde-Rowan, M. D., Rekate, H. L., Nulsen, F. E. (1982) 'Reexpansion of previously collapsed ventricles: the slit ventricle syndrome.' *Journal of Neurosurgery,* **56,** 536-539.
Knake, J. E., Chandler, W. F., McGillicuddy, J. E., Silver, T. M., Gabrielsen, T. O. (1982) 'Intraoperative sonography for brain tumor localization and ventricular shunt placement.' *American Journal of Roentgenology,* **139,** 733-738 (see also: *American Journal of Neuroradiology,* **3,** 425-430).
Levene, M. I. (1982) 'Ventricular tap under direct ultrasound control.' *Archives of Disease in Childhood,* **57,** 873-875.
Scotti, G., Musgrave, M. A., Fitz, C. R., Harwood-Nash, D. C. (1980) 'The isolated fourth ventricle in

children: CT and clinical review of 16 cases.' *American Journal of Roentgenology,* **135,** 1233-1238 (see also: *American Journal of Neuroradiology,* **1,** 419-424).

Shkolnik, A., McLone, D. G. (1981) 'Intraoperative real-time ultrasonic guidance of ventricular shunt placement in infants.' *Radiology,* **141,** 515-517.

—— —— (1982) 'Intraoperative real-time ultrasonic guidance of intracranial shunt tube placement in infants.' *Radiology,* **144,** 573-576.

Yamada, H., Nakamura, S., Tanaka, Y., Tajima, M., Kageyama, N. (1982) 'Ventriculography and cisternography with water soluble contrast media in infants with myelomengocele.' *Radiology,* **143,** 75-83.

12
ULTRASOUND OF THE SPINE

Until the age of eight to 12 months of life, the posterior elements of the bony spine are poorly ossified, and ultrasound imaging of the spinal cord is possible (Schieble *et al.* 1983). An operative defect (laminectomy) or congenital dysraphism (myelomeningocele) produces larger bone and cartilage-free portals for imaging (Braun *et al.* 1983).

Standard real-time or static scanners can be used to produce satisfactory images. A 5 or 7MHz transducer is adequate, although ranges up to 10MHz have been reported (Schieble *et al.* 1983). The lower-range transducer (5MHz) is best employed with some form of water-path or stand-off device. A water-filled latex examination glove works very well, and places the spinal cord well within the focal plane of the transducer. Static, real-time and automated water-path scanning devices (Miller *et al.* 1982) can readily obtain both axial and sagittal ultrasound images.

Meningoceles, myelomeningoceles and lipomyelomeningoceles are protruding soft tissue masses found posteriorly, usually in the lumbar spine. Clinically, a sac contains neural elements when symptoms such as neurogenic bowel and/or bladder dysfunction, flaccid paralysis and sensory deficits are present. Hair tufts, dimples or sinuses, haemangiomas, lipomas, pigmented naevi, kyphosis or focal scoliosis may be present at the site of the lesion. These may even be found in the absence of any

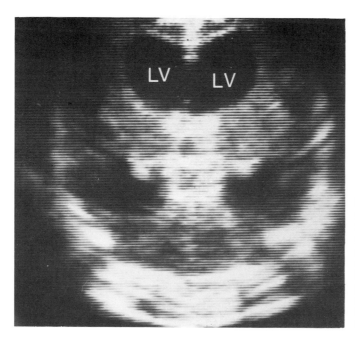

Fig. 12.1. Hydrocephalus associated with meningocele. Coronal sonogram shows moderate ventricular enlargement of lateral ventricles (LV). Unilocular lumbar meningocele was present and ventricular enlargement was not suspected. A renal ultrasound examination was normal.

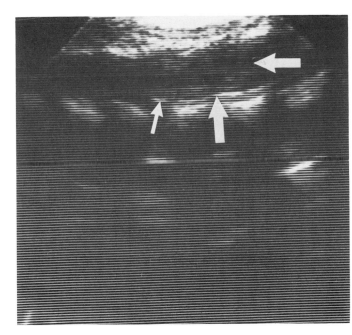

Fig. 12.2. Normal sagittal sonogram of the spine. Longitudinal image demonstrates normal low-level echoes rising from spinal cord and nerve roots *(right arrow)*. The strongly reflective vertebral bodies produce regular echoes *(left arrows)* with transmission through intervertebral disc spaces.

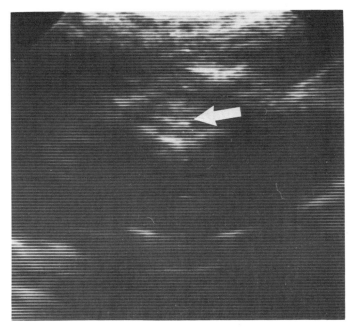

Fig. 12.3. Normal axial sonogram of the spine. Little attenuation is produced by cartilage of posterior elements in this axial scan of a neonate. Normal faint spinal cord echoes are seen *(arrow)* with no visualisation of small central canal.

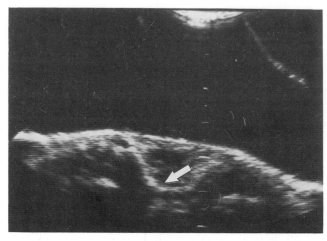

Fig. 12.4. Decompressed meningocele. An axial sonogram, performed through a water-filled latex glove, shows abnormal fluid accumulation *(arrow)* within neural tube. Elevation of head of cot will occasionally cause meningocele to bulge slightly and become more prominent.

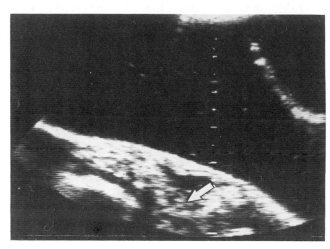

Fig. 12.5. Lipomeningocele. A longitudinal or sagittal sonogram shows abnormally increased echogenicity of spinal cord *(arrow)* just proximal to the small dorsal defect. At surgery, this proved to be a lipoma of the cord.

neurological signs (Green 1980).

Infants and young children with a lumbar mass should also have a renal ultrasound examination in order to identify possible hydronephrosis. There is a high association with intracranial ventricular dilatation (Fig. 12.1) and a cranial ultrasound examination should also be performed (Babcock and Han 1980, Yamada *et al.* 1982).

The normal spine produces varying degrees of acoustical shadowing. More complete shadowing is seen anterior to the spinal cord, arising from the more heavily calcified vertebral bodies (Fig. 12.2). The regular and repetitive appearance of the bony spinal elements is quite constant on longitudinal images. The spinal cord is a regular collection of low-level echoes with a somewhat prominent posterior and anterior wall (Fig. 12.3), arising from the cerebrospinal fluid (CSF) interface (Miller *et al.* 1982, Schieble *et al.* 1983). Rapid tapering at the termination of the cord is found at the L3 level in infants and up to the L1-L2 level in older children. The central canal of the cord is usually not seen with lower-frequency transducers.

The filum terminale is a more prominent echogenic band that extends down from the conus. Both it and the cord should pulsate gently on real-time examination. In the infant, non-motion or fixation of the filum terminale and cord strongly suggests tethering, even in the absence of clinical symptoms (Heinz *et al.* 1979, Raghavendra *et al.* 1983).

A meningocele contains only CSF and no neural elements (Fig. 12.4). The sac is clearly cystic and occasionally communicates directly with the extra-axial space. Unfortunately, plaques or linear collections of dysplastic neural tissue are sometimes seen on the wall of a meningocele (Jacobs *et al.* 1984). This makes the distinction between a simple meningocele and a complex myelomeningocele more difficult. Multi-loculated sacs are sometimes found and almost always contain nerve roots. Myelomeningoceles may be unilocular but always contain nerve roots as well (Miller *et al.* 1982). Open or draining meningocele sacs can be examined with care. Sterile gels or flowing solutions should be used as the coupling agent. Enclosing the transducer in a sterile cover prevents contamination of the defect.

Solid tumours are rare and may be intradural or extradural (Fig. 12.5). An echogenic soft tissue mass deforming or displacing the weakly echogenic cord are the principal signs (Braun *et al.* 1983). Hydromelia is represented by intrathecal unilocular anechoic masses arising from the central canal. A multiseptated mass in or on the cord suggests an arteriovenous malformation or cavernous haemangioma. Prominent pulsations in such a vascular mass, while expected, may not be present.

Tissue characterization of spinal lesions by ultrasound is important though not critical prior to surgical therapy. Tethering of the spinal cord can be demonstrated on a pre-operative ultrasound examination. In addition, the size of a lipoma or teratoma within a myelomeningocele is helpful pre-operative information (Miller *et al.* 1982).

REFERENCES

Braun, I. F., Raghavendra, B. N., Kricheff, I. I. (1983) 'Spinal cord imaging using real-time high-resolution ultrasound.' *Radiology,* **147,** 459-465.
Green, M. (1980) *Pediatric Diagnosis, 3rd Edn.* Philadelphia: W. B. Saunders. pp. 192-194.
Heinz, E. R., Rosenbaum, A. E., Scarff, T. B., Reigel, D. H., Drayer, B. P. (1979) 'Tethered spinal cord following meningomyelocele repair.' *Radiology,* **131,** 153-160.
Jacobs, N. M., Grant, E. G., Dagi, T. F., Richardson, J. D. (1984) 'Ultrasound identification of neural elements in myelomeningocele.' *Journal of Clinical Ultrasound,* **12,** 51-53.
Miller, J. H., Reid, B. S.,, Kemberling, C. R. (1982) 'Utilization of ultrasound in the evaluation of spinal dysraphism in children.' *Radiology,* **143,** 737-740.
Raghavendra, B. N., Epstein, F. J., Pinto, R. S., Subramanyam, B. R., Greenberg, J., Mitnick, J. S. (1983) 'The tethered spinal cord: diagnosis by high-resolution real-time ultrasound.' *Radiology,* **149,** 123-128.
Schieble, W., James, H. E., Leopold, G. R., Hilton, S. W. (1983) 'Occult spinal dysraphism in infants: screening with high-resolution real-time ultrasound.' *Radiology,* **146,** 743-746.
Yamada, H., Nakamura, S., Tanaka, Y., Tajima, M., Kageyama, N. (1982) 'Ventriculography and cisternography with water-soluble contrast media in infants with myelomeningocele.' *Radiology,* **143,** 75-83.

13
ULTRASOUND AND OTHER IMAGING TECHNIQUES

In this book we have attempted to show the versatility of ultrasound in the investigation of newborn intracranial pathology, and the number of chapters attests to its value in this area. We have noted that ultrasound may not always be the best technique to exclude or confidently diagnose a particular pathological process or congenital abnormality. In the area of periventricular haemorrhage there is little doubt that high resolution real-time sector ultrasound scanning is currently the best technique. Its correlation with autopsy data is excellent. Portable ultrasound equipment permits convenient and safe scanning of an infant in the intensive care unit, and makes it a useful device for intracranial imaging even for those conditions in which it is not totally reliable. If, however, the infant is well enough to travel to the radiology department, then other imaging techniques may be utilised.

Apart from the detection of a skull fracture or a bony abnormality, there is little place for a plain skull film in infants. Intracranial pathology is much more amenable to other forms of investigation. Recognition of the level of obstruction in hydrocephalus, and identification of a connection between the ventricle and a porencephalic cyst, may be important prior to a shunting procedure. In these circumstances, radionuclide or contrast encephalography may be the most appropriate investigation.

The introduction of radiographic computerised tomography (CT) revolutionised the approach to brain imaging. Computerised tomography gives complete cross-sectional images at a number of levels with superior resolution. Ultrasound visualisation is limited in the extreme frontal and occipital poles as well as in the most lateral parietal regions. Consequently, small subarachnoid and subdural haemorrhages may be missed on ultrasound examination, but can be detected with CT. The posterior fossa may not be well visualised by ultrasound, nor by CT. The diagnosis of intercerebellar haemorrhage may be missed using either modality.

Ultrasound has advantages over CT in that it does not utilise ionizing radiation, and the infant rarely requires sedation prior to the examination. Sonography may be more sensitive than CT in detecting small areas of calcification (see Chapter 10). As the ventricles can be scanned in real-time, maximum dimensions can be measured and small deviations in shape can be appreciated; this is not possible with CT. Periventricular leukomalacia is more amenable to detection by sonography, particularly in the early stages when cystic degeneration is just beginning to occur (Chapter 6). Congenital abnormalities of the brain are also easily recognised by ultrasound examination.

Infants with areas of abnormally increased echodensity in the cerebral parenchyma may be assumed to have a haemorrhagic lesion. However, it may be

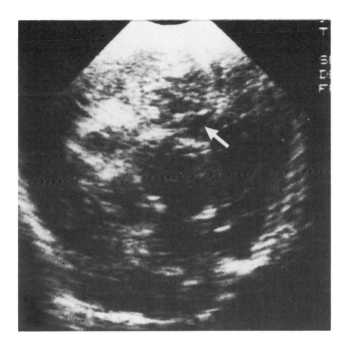

Fig. 13.1. Coronal ultrasound scan showing diffuse echogenic areas in left hemisphere causing distortion of right lateral ventricle *(arrow)* and deviation of midline structures.

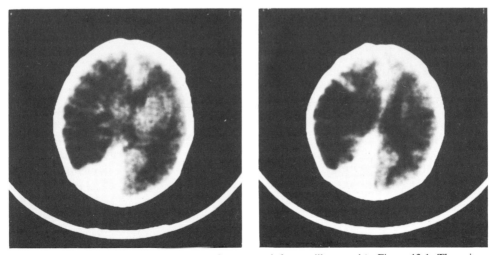

Fig. 13.2. Computerised X-ray tomograms from same infant as illustrated in Figure 13.1. There is an obvious wedge-shaped infarct of posterior cerebral artery together with extensive oedema involving right hemisphere.

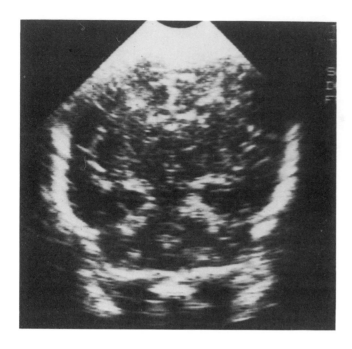

Fig. 13.3. Ultrasound scan from infant suffering from severe birth asphyxia. There is no obvious abnormality.

difficult to make a distinction between haemorrhage, haemorrhagic venous infarction and arterial infarction. Figure 13.1 shows a large parenchymal 'haemorrhage' diagnosed by ultrasound in a full-term infant. A CT scan showed the classical wedge-shaped pattern of arterial infarction (Fig. 13.2). Neonatal 'stroke' diagnosed by CT (Mannino and Trauner 1983) has been described in the literature. It is advisable to consider obtaining a CT scan in any infant born at term with apparent primary parenchymal haemorrhage.

The diagnosis of cerebral oedema may be difficult to make by CT, particularly in preterm infants. Comparison of CT and ultrasound in term asphyxiated babies confirms that CT may show marked abnormalities in infants with normal ultrasound scans (Figs. 13.3 and 13.4). In the premature infant with cerebral oedema, neither technique is particularly reliable (Flodmark *et al.* 1980). In addition, the infant with dilated ventricles may present a diagnostic problem in differentiating between high- and low-pressure hydrocephalus, or in excluding ventriculomegaly secondary to atrophy.

Recently, nuclear magnetic resonance (NMR) imaging has been used in the newborn to investigate intracranial structure and pathology (Levene *et al.* 1982*a*). NMR relies on the paramagnetic properties of the hydrogen proton to generate an image. The head is placed within a strong homogeneous magnetic field and perturbation of the protons induced by a radio-frequency impulse. Relaxation times of the protons are detected by the same radio-frequency coil, and this information can be mathematically converted to a tomographic image. In addition to producing anatomical images, NMR is particularly useful in detecting myelin-

142

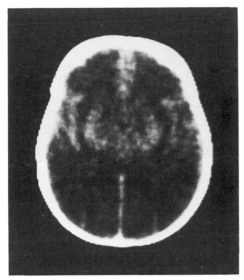

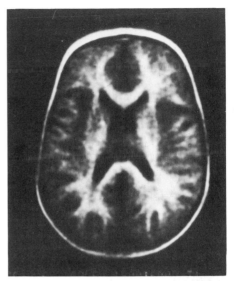

Fig. 13.4. Computerised X-ray tomogram from patient as illustrated in Figure 13.3. There are marked areas of low attenuation consistent with cerebral oedema.

Fig. 13.5. Nuclear magnetic resonance (NMR) scan in axial section (T1 dependent image) showing myelination as white areas extending anteriorly (forceps minor) and posteriorly (forceps major) as well as being present in internal capsule. (Reproduced by permission of the editor of the British Medical Journal.)

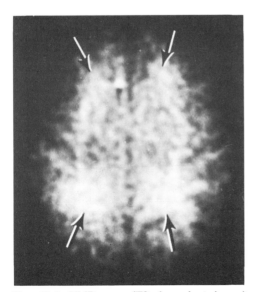

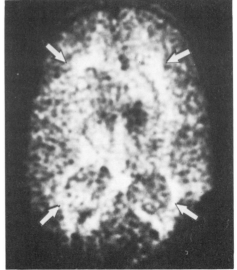

Fig. 13.6. NMR scan (T2 dependent image) showing white areas *(arrowed)* consistent with cerebral oedema. (Reproduced by permission of the editor of the British Medical Journal.)

Fig. 13.7. NMR scan (T2 dependent image) showing white (short T2) areas *(arrowed)* consistent with periventricular oedema. (Reproduced by permission of the editor of the British Medical Journal.)

ation, intracerebral water (Levene *et al.* 1982*b*), and other abnormalities (Johnson *et al.* 1983). No other imaging technique has the ability to demonstrate myelination (Fig. 13.5), and this may be important in the assessment of recovery from perinatal insults. In infants with severe birth asphyxia, NMR scans reveal diffuse areas in the periventricular regions, indicating cerebral oedema (Fig. 13.6). Acute hydrocephalus shows lighter areas at the margins of dilated lateral ventricles (Fig. 13.7). This probably reflects transependymal fluid exudate, which was not seen on a CT scan.

The rôle for NMR in cranial imaging of the infant is not yet defined, although it has considerable potential and may eventually be preferred to CT. By using alternative imaging modalities, mechanical and physiological limitations of ultrasound scanning may be avoided. Currently, ultrasound scanning is the initial technique of choice to image the infant's brain with suspected intracranial pathology.

REFERENCES

Flodmark, O., Becker, L. E., Harwood-Nash, D. L., Fitzhardinge, P. M., Fitz, C. R., Chuang, S. H. (1980) 'Correlation between computed tomography and autopsy in premature and full-term neonates that have suffered perinatal asphyxia.' *Radiology, 137,* 93-103.
Johnson, M. A., Pennock, J. M., Bydder, G. M., Steiner, R. E., Thomas, D. J., Haywood, R., Bryant, D. K. T., Payne, J. A., Levene, M. I., Whitelaw, A., Dubowitz, L. M. S., Dubowitz, V. (1983) 'Clinical NMR imaging of the brain of children: normal and neurologic disease.' *American Journal of Neuroradiology, 4,* 1013-26.
Levene, M. I., Whitelaw, A., Dubowitz, L. M. S., Dubowitz, V., Bydder, G. M., Steiner, R. E. (1982*a*) 'Nuclear magnetic resonance imaging of IVH and related disorders.' *Second Special Ross Laboratories Conference on Perinatal Intracranial Hemorrhage Syllabus, 1,* 595-613.
—— —— Dubowitz, V., Bydder, G. M., Steiner, R. E., Randall, C. P., Young, I. R. (1982*b*) 'Nuclear magnetic resonance imaging of the brain of children.' *British Medical Journal, 285,* 774-776.
Mannino, F. L., Trauner, D. A. (1983) 'Stroke in neonates.' *Journal of Pediatrics, 102,* 605-610.

INDEX